The Beginner's Guide to Keto Diet for Meat Lovers, Vegetarians, and Vegans

Perfect How-to Guide for Onboarding the Ketogenic Lifestyle Including Meal Plans for Weight Loss, Vitality, and Well-Being

Paul Lawrence

© Copyright 2021 - All rights reserved.

The content contained within this book may not be reproduced, duplicated or transmitted without direct written permission from the author or the publisher.

Under no circumstances will any blame or legal responsibility be held against the publisher, or author, for any damages, reparation, or monetary loss due to the information contained within this book, either directly or indirectly.

Legal Notice:

This book is copyright protected. It is only for personal use. You cannot amend, distribute, sell, use, quote or paraphrase any part, or the content within this book, without the consent of the author or publisher.

Disclaimer Notice:

Please note the information contained within this document is for educational and entertainment purposes only. All effort has been executed to present accurate, up to date, reliable, complete information. No warranties of any kind are declared or implied. Readers acknowledge that the author is not engaged in the rendering of legal, financial, medical or professional advice. The content within this book has been derived from various sources. Please consult a licensed professional before attempting any techniques outlined in this book.

By reading this document, the reader agrees that under no circumstances is the author responsible for any losses, direct or indirect, that are incurred as a result of the use of the information contained within this document, including, but not limited to, errors, omissions, or inaccuracies.

Table of Contents

INTRODUCTION 1

CHAPTER 1: THE SCIENCE BEHIND THE MAGICAL EFFECTS OF KETOSIS 3

   HOW FOOD IS TURNED INTO ENERGY 3
   KETOSIS 4
   THE KETO DIET HAS MANY HEALTH BENEFITS 5
      Epilepsy 6
      Certain Cancers 6
      Autism 7
      Polycystic Ovary Syndrome (PCOS) 7
      Glucose Transporter 1 (GLUT1) Deficiency Syndrome 7
      Diabetes 8
      Migraines 8
      Multiple Sclerosis (MS) 8

CHAPTER 2: ADOPTING THE KETO LIFESTYLE 11

   SOME THINGS WORTH CONSIDERING 12
      Get to Know What Foods to Eat and What to Avoid 13
      Take Note of the Downsides of a Keto diet 19
      You Might Experience Some Nutrient Deficiencies 20
   KETO TIPS AND TRICKS 21
      Who Should Steer Clear of the Keto Diet? 21
      To Get Started 22
      As a Beginner, Consider Other Methods of the Keto Diet 23
   11 FREQUENTLY ASKED QUESTIONS 24

CHAPTER 3: INTERMITTENT FASTING 27

   THE BENEFITS OF INTERMITTENT FASTING 28
      It Can Alter the Function of Genes, Hormones, and Cells 29
      It Can Lower Your Risk of Type 2 Diabetes 30
      It Can Reduce Inflammation and Oxidative Stress in the Body 30
      It May Be Beneficial for Heart Health 30
      It May Extend Your Lifespan 31
   COMBINING THE KETO DIET WITH INTERMITTENT FASTING 31

CHAPTER 4: A 14-DAY MEAL PLAN WITH RECIPES FOR MEAT EATERS 33

DAY 1 35
   Breakfast (Optional): Traditional Keto Coffee 35
   Lunch: Creamy Salmon and Zucchini Pasta 36
   Dinner: One-Pot Chicken and Broccoli Delight... 38
DAY 2 39
   Breakfast (Optional): Creamy Coconut Coffee.. 39
   Lunch: Spanish Omelet 40
   Dinner: Sautéed Vegetables With Lemony Garlic Salmon 41
DAY 3 43
   Breakfast (Optional): Bacon and Chicken Sausages 43
   Lunch: Baked Egg in Avocado (a keto favorite) 44
   Dinner: Potato less Cottage Pie 46
DAY 4 47
   Breakfast: Easy Keto Frittatas 47
   Lunch: Chicken and Zucchini Noodle Soup... 49
   Dinner: Sesame Beef Teriyaki and Kale.. 50
DAY 5 51
   Breakfast (Optional): Zucchini Bread 51
   Lunch: Pan-Fried Turkey, Bacon, and Vegetables 53
   Dinner: Spicy Keto Chili 54
DAY 6 56
   Breakfast (Optional): Chocolate Hazelnut Muffins.................................... 56
   Lunch: Lemony Pepper Tuna Salad 57
   Dinner: Apple Dijon Pork Chops (serve with broccoli if desired) 58
DAY 7 60
   Breakfast (Optional): Frothy Bulletproof Coffee 60
   Lunch: Caesar Salad With Garlic Shrimp.. 61
   Dinner: Pan-Fried Pork Tenderloin With Garlic Spinach 62
DAY 8 64
   Breakfast (Optional): Breakfast Stack 64
   Lunch: Chicken Cauliflower Couscous Salad 65
   Dinner: Super Easy Salmon Curry... 66
DAY 9 68
   Breakfast (Optional): Blueberry Muffins... 68
   Lunch: Mini Ham and Spinach Quiches... 70
   Dinner: Beef Fajitas.. 71
DAY 10 72
   Breakfast (Optional): Collagen Booster Coffee 72
   Lunch: Mini Spinach Meatloaves 73
   Dinner: Creamy Tomato and Chicken Keto Pasta 75
DAY 11 76
   Breakfast (Optional): Apple Cinnamon Muffins... 76

Lunch: Bacon and Avo Caesar Salad *77*
Dinner: Pork and Cabbage Stew *79*
DAY 12 81
Breakfast (Optional): Yummy French Pancakes *81*
Lunch: Smoked Salmon Ham Wraps With Cucumber *83*
Dinner: Roast Beef With Carrots and Onions *84*
DAY 13 85
Breakfast: Eggs Benedict With Mug Bread *85*
Lunch: Blueberry Chaffels *88*
Dinner: Cheesy Meatballs (Italian Style) *89*
DAY 14 91
Breakfast: Classic Bacon and Eggs *91*
Lunch: Seafood Chowder *92*
Dinner: Bacon and Mushroom Casserole *93*

CHAPTER 5: A 12-DAY MEAL PLAN WITH RECIPES FOR VEGETARIANS 95

DAY 1 96
Breakfast (Optional): Strawberry Smoothie *96*
Lunch: Delicious Deviled Eggs *97*
Dinner: Goat Cheese and Spinach Pie *98*
DAY 2 100
Breakfast (Optional): Buttery Basil Scrambled Eggs *100*
Lunch: Cauliflower Hash Browns *102*
Dinner: Homemade Pesto Gnocchi *103*
DAY 3 105
Breakfast (Optional): Easy Mexican-Style Eggs *105*
Lunch: A Simple Greek Salad *107*
Dinner: Rich and Creamy Broccoli and Leek Soup *109*
DAY 4 111
Breakfast (Optional): Blueberry Smoothie *111*
Lunch: Swedish Turnip Fritters *112*
Dinner: Garlic Bread *114*
DAY 5 116
Breakfast (Optional): Cranberry and Kale Salad *116*
Lunch: Tortilla Pizzas *119*
Dinner: Grilled Portobello "Steaks" *120*
DAY 6 122
Breakfast (Optional): Crispy Sesame Bread *122*
Lunch: Goat Cheese Salad With Balsamic Vinegar *124*
Dinner: Vegetarian Tapas *125*
DAY 7 127
Breakfast (Optional): Avocado Smoothie *127*

Lunch: Stuffed Zucchini Skins 128
Dinner: Cheesy Ratatouille 130
DAY 8 132
Breakfast (Optional): Spinach and Feta Crustless Quiche 132
Lunch: Cured and Marinated Halloumi Bites 133
Dinner: Roasted Onion and Cauliflower Soup 135
DAY 9 136
Breakfast (Optional): Pancake Cereal 136
Lunch: Easy Warm Egg Salad 138
Dinner: Curry Bake 140
DAY 10 142
Breakfast (Optional): Caprese Paninis 142
Lunch: Savory Veggie Loaf 144
Dinner: Mushroom and Ricotta Galette 145
DAY 11 148
Breakfast (Optional): English Veggie Bowl 148
Lunch: Jalapeño Cheese Bread 150
Dinner: Roasted "Potatoes" With Garlic and Feta 151
DAY 12 153
Breakfast (Optional): Caprese Omelet 153
Lunch: Roasted Pumpkin Salad 155
Dinner: Baked Italian Mushrooms 156

CHAPTER 6: A 7-DAY MEAL PLAN WITH RECIPES FOR VEGANS **158**
DAY 1 159
Breakfast (Optional): Grilled Harissa Eggplant 159
Lunch: The Immune Booster Soup 160
Dinner: Superfood Salad Bowl 162
DAY 2 164
Breakfast (Optional): Strawberry and Rhubarb Smoothie 164
Lunch: Easy Tomato Salad 165
Dinner: Asian Spiced Broccoli 166
DAY 3 168
Breakfast (Optional): Stuffed Avocado 168
Lunch: Minty Zucchini Salad 169
Dinner: Spicy Vegetable Curry 171
DAY 4 173
Breakfast (Optional): Blueberry and Lemon Electrolyte Drink 173
Lunch: Cabbage, Avocado, and Almond Salad 174
Dinner: Braised Fennel With Lemon 176
DAY 5 177
Breakfast (Optional): Pumpkin Spice Latte 177

Lunch: Sesame Carrot Falafel 178
  Dinner: Vegan Tikka Masala 180
 DAY 6 182
  Breakfast (Optional): Cinnamon and Pecan Porridge 182
  Lunch: Lemony Garlic Roasted Broccoli 184
  Dinner: Pesto Zoodles (Zucchini Noodles) 186
 DAY 7 187
  Breakfast (Optional): Dairy-Free Ketoccino 187
  Lunch: Spicy Zucchini Chips 189
  Dinner: Spinach and Mushroom Soup 190

CONCLUSION **192**

REFERENCES **194**
 IMAGES 208

Introduction

The ketogenic diet has taken the world by storm in recent years and with good reason. It has proved its worth through the many success stories that have been reported. We live in times where many diets have been tried, and some may even say that none of these famous diets have had quite the effect that the ketogenic diet has.

With all this fame comes numerous controversies, though. It seems quite impossible that a low-carb, high-fat diet could be more beneficial than it is harmful, and that's understandable. We've grown up believing that fat is the devil and that we need whole grains and fruit to boost our energy levels. Recent studies have proven otherwise.

One of the controversies that have made its rounds is the fact that our bodies need carbohydrates to function efficiently. While this is true for professional athletes, it's not the case for people who live normal lives. There is no high-quality research that suggests taking in a decent amount of carbs in the form of whole grains, such as bread and pasta, will protect us from disease or prolong our lives. However, although fewer carbs are recommended, they do not get cut from the keto diet completely.

"Won't I suffer from a nutrient deficiency if I give up whole grains and fruit?" I hear you ask. You're more likely to improve your nutrient intake by substituting these carbs with vegetables that are lower in carbohydrates but higher in nutritional value. Flour, bread, and pasta do not contain specific nutrients that our bodies need. The modern fruit that we buy has been genetically modified to taste sweet. Except for vitamin C, fruit really does not offer as many vitamins and minerals as you might think. Blending handfuls of fruit into smoothies every day only boosts your sugar levels and offers minimal health-related benefits.

It is also widely believed that our brains need carbs to function even though they can be fueled by fat. You might think that this diet is not for you because you don't eat meat or suffer from kidney disease. Consuming fat does not mean that you have to consume protein, and this seems to be a common misconception. There are many ways to consume fat without having to add red meat (or any meat for that matter) to your diet.

We have been at war with fat for a long time. Low-fat foods have been flying off the shelves for years, skim milk has become popular, and butter has become frowned upon. This book aims to change your mindset toward the low-carb, high-fat controversy that we have been programmed to believe is unhealthy. We'll talk about why you should start buying butter again; opt for organic, full-fat milk; and steer clear of low-fat labels.

Our bodies undergo ketosis daily regardless of the number of carbs that we consume. Most people are never in ketosis due to the high-protein and high-carb diets that they are so familiar with, and our bodies prefer sugar as a primary source of fuel. If you've ever skipped a meal, your body has experienced a mild level of ketosis. It's important to understand how ketosis works before you jump on the keto train!

So, are you ready to get started on your keto journey? Everything you need and more can be found in this book and at my website, www.3in1keto.com. Let's go!

Chapter 1:

The Science Behind the Magical Effects of Ketosis

Since the body prefers sugar as its primary source of fuel, we have gotten so used to filling up on carbohydrates to maintain our energy throughout the long days that we have been forced to grow accustomed to it. We work long hours and look forward to the guilty pleasures of fast food and sweet treats to reward ourselves for our hard work every day. We don't think about what we're putting into our bodies during the day. Instead, we comfort ourselves by thinking that we deserve chocolate after putting up with a difficult boss all day. We're so busy earning a living, taking care of kids, or maintaining a home that we feel we simply don't have the time to cook healthy meals.

To understand the process of ketosis, it's imperative to understand how the body turns food into energy first. By understanding how this works, we might think twice about opting for unhealthy food choices. Understanding how your body works is the first step toward making better choices. Not only for the sake of losing weight but also to live a healthier lifestyle that will improve your quality of life.

How Food Is Turned Into Energy

After a meal, our body digests the food we just ate. The hefty amount of carbohydrates from the bread or slice of cake we ate is broken down into glucose (sugar) and then released into the bloodstream. Insulin, a hormone responsible for driving glucose into cell tissue, then sends the glucose in your bloodstream to the cells to store as fuel for later use. Insulin opens the cell doors to let glucose in. Without insulin, glucose will remain in the bloodstream, causing high blood sugar levels (hyperglycemia). If there are large amounts of glucose in your bloodstream as a result of the number of carbohydrates (sugar and starches) you've consumed, insulin production increases.

So, where does insulin come from? It's produced by the beta cells in the pancreas, and these cells are extremely sensitive to the amount of glucose in your bloodstream. Your body automatically checks your glucose levels as often as every few seconds and can determine when insulin production needs to be increased or decreased. The rise and fall of blood sugar levels and insulin happens regularly through the day and night. The balance of the right amounts of insulin to control glucose levels is the secret to maintaining our energy to live and function.

Ketosis

Exercising for longer than an hour, skipping a meal, or limiting carbohydrates is how ketosis can be kickstarted. We've all experienced mild ketosis before, but we don't allow our bodies to take full advantage of it!

When there's a lack of carbohydrates to digest and turn into sugar, ketone production increases. Ketones are highly efficient energy molecules that come from fat stores. To meet your brain's need for energy, the fat gets broken down into fatty acids and glycerol. The fatty acids and glycerol then enter the liver where they're converted into sugar. This process might sound familiar, but you probably thought that only carbs could be converted into sugar, right?

Furthermore, the glycerol is converted into glucose (a process called gluconeogenesis) and the fatty acids into ketone bodies (ketogenesis). As a result of ketogenesis, ketone bodies produce acetoacetate, which is then broken down into two other types of ketone bodies: beta-hydroxybutyrate (BHB) and acetone. Acetone can be turned into glucose but is mostly excreted as waste, whereas BHB is a more efficient source of fuel than glucose. The brain and body prefer BHB and acetoacetate as a source of fuel because they're 70% more efficient for cells than glucose.

Our bodies can't rely on ketosis alone as a source of fuel, which is why gluconeogenesis is necessary. I've already mentioned how the liver can divert glycerol (a fat component) into glucose, but the amino acids from protein and lactate from muscle can be converted into sugar as well, which goes to show that your body is capable of producing its own sugar. We've got our liver to thank for that; it constantly meets the glucose needs of the brain and body, even if we restrict our carb intake or skip a meal.

Even though ketogenesis and gluconeogenesis team up to work together when carbohydrates are limited, you can get in the way of ketones being steadily increased. If you consume too much protein, for example, your body will increase gluconeogenesis and restrict ketosis. This is because ketone production and insulin levels are linked. Too much protein may increase the need for insulin, which downregulates ketogenesis. This is why protein consumption on the keto diet is moderate; you should consume enough protein to maintain muscle mass but not so much that it limits your body's ability to experience ketosis.

The Keto Diet Has Many Health Benefits

The keto diet has a reputation for its weight-loss benefits. Surprisingly, few know of its health benefits. Cutting carbs is one of the most effective ways to lose weight; it aids in lowering insulin levels and rids the body of excess water. You won't be hungry all the time since low-carb diets automatically decrease your appetite. People who cut carbs eat more protein and fat, yet they don't consume a lot of calories (Fj et al, 2007). Studies have shown that people on low-carb diets lose weight faster than those on low-fat diets, even if the latter were restricting calories.

New research suggests that following the ketogenic diet can improve your quality of life and even aid in simplifying the management of some diseases.

Epilepsy

The keto diet has been shown to reduce the amount of glutamate (neurotransmitters responsible for sending signals between nerve cells) in the brain. It also increases the amount of gamma-aminobutyric acid (GABA), which is responsible for producing a calming effect after it attaches to a protein in the brain. Since this diet reduces inflammation in the brain, the chances of a seizure occurring are reduced significantly. Studies show that the keto diet reduces the number of seizures by 50% in half of the patients. This is because ketones cross the blood-brain barrier of the brain and are used as an alternative source of energy by the brain when glucose levels have been reduced. According to D'Andrea Meira et al (2019), the keto diet mimics the fasting state, causing the body to use fats as a primary source of fuel. The ketogenic diet may even improve numerous brain patterns regardless of seizure control.

Certain Cancers

Even though it is not suggested that cancer patients use the keto diet as a stand-alone treatment, it can be used in combination with chemotherapy and radiation. A study has shown that cancer cells may be less likely to grow if the body uses fat as a source of fuel instead of glucose (Zick et al, 2018). This is because the ketogenic diet lowers insulin levels as a result of lower blood sugar, which aids in preventing tumor growth. Several case studies on the effects of the ketogenic diet on tumor metabolism found improvements in glioblastoma multiforme (GBM), one of the most aggressive forms of brain cancer, and various other types of brain cancer.

Autism

Usually diagnosed in childhood, autism spectrum disorder (ASD) shares similarities with epilepsy since it can cause overactive brain cells, which can result in a seizure. This condition is characterized by issues with communication, social interaction, and, sometimes, repetitive behaviors. Studies in mice and rats showed improvement in behaviors related to ASD as the keto diet reduced the over-stimulation of brain cells. A pilot study on the application of a ketogenic diet in children with autism that involved 30 children found that 18 of them showed improvement in symptoms after following the ketogenic diet for six months (Evangeliou et al, 2003).

Polycystic Ovary Syndrome (PCOS)

PCOS is a hormonal imbalance that causes cysts to grow on the ovaries, causing irregular periods and, sometimes, infertility. Usually, women with PCOS are obese because one of its characteristics is insulin resistance. Women with PCOS are at risk of developing type 2 diabetes, and they may have trouble losing weight. A pilot study on the effects of the keto diet in women with PCOS in which 11 women followed a ketogenic diet showed an average of 12% in weight loss. This study also found that their fasting insulin levels decreased by as much as 54%, and their fertility hormone production increased. Two of them suffered from infertility but managed to become pregnant (Mavropoulos et al, 2005).

Glucose Transporter 1 (GLUT1) Deficiency Syndrome

GLUT1 deficiency syndrome is a rare genetic disorder that involves the deficiency of a unique protein responsible for sending glucose to the brain. Symptoms usually start as early as just after birth and include a delay in development, movement difficulty, and, in some cases, seizures. Since the ketogenic diet provides fat as a source of fuel instead of glucose, the transportation of fuel to the brain is possible.

Ketones do not require this protein to cross through the blood barrier of the brain. In a study on the effects of the keto diet in children with this protein deficiency, it was found that seizure occurrences decreased. Muscle coordination, concentration, and alertness in these children improved.

Diabetes

The ketogenic diet has been shown to significantly reduce blood sugar levels in people with type 1 and type 2 diabetes. In a study that took place over 16 weeks, 17 people out of 21 were able to decrease their diabetes medication dosages on the ketogenic diet. Some were even able to discontinue their medication. Study participants managed to lose an average of 19 pounds, and their waist size reduced as well as their blood pressure and triglycerides (a major form of fat stored by the body). The same study found that hemoglobin A1c (glycated hemoglobin, a form of hemoglobin chemically linked to sugar) in diabetic patients reduced after a year of following the ketogenic diet, more so than patients who followed a low-fat, calorie-restricted diet.

Migraines

A migraine is not your typical headache. A migraine has symptoms of light sensitivity, severe pain, and extreme nausea. Even though more studies are needed to prove the results of following a ketogenic diet and its effects on migraines, there has been some evidence that suggests that the keto diet may reduce the frequency and symptoms of migraines. An observational study reported the reduction in the use of pain medication after one month of following the keto diet.

Multiple Sclerosis (MS)

MS is a disease that damages nerves, causing problems with the communication process between the body and the brain. Symptoms include problems with memory, vision, balance, and movement. As with other nervous system diseases, MS seems to reduce the cells' ability to use glucose as a source of fuel. A review suggested that patients who followed a low-carb, high-fat diet showed an improvement in cell tissue repair because of the keto diet's potential assistance with energy production. A study involving MS in mice found that the keto diet actually reduced inflammation, improving physical function and memory.

By now, you're probably wondering how and where to start. Not only does the keto diet offer many health benefits, but it's also fairly easy to get started. It only requires a little determination, a positive mindset, and a few tips and tricks to guide you on your journey.

Chapter 2:

Adopting the Keto Lifestyle

The convenience of processed foods has led to an increase in obesity-related diseases such as heart disease, type 2 diabetes, and kidney disease, to name a few. Man-made foods are sending the health of many on a downward spiral because they are affordable, easy to consume (most processed foods don't require cooking; it's a matter of heat and eat), and so readily available! We have given up the nutritious foods that contain natural sources of fiber and vitamins necessary to prolong our lives and improve our quality of life. Pre-diabetes is on the rise, increasing the risk of developing type 2 diabetes.

We're constantly on the go, juggling work, family time, and free time to the point where we don't have the time to cook decent meals anymore. Fast foods have become the new normal, and we don't think twice before gulping down a large soda. There are three main problems with our modern-day diet:

1. Our sugar intake has dramatically increased. From an evolutionary perspective, whole foods that contain natural sugar were seasonal. Since then, nutrients have become so refined that we are left with corn syrup and fructose. These are the culprits contributing to obesity, metabolic syndrome, type 2 diabetes, and cardiovascular disease. Then came the low-fat craze; the food industry started processing natural fats out of many foods, replacing them with sugar to make food palatable and to use it as a preservative. As a result, the shelf life of food has increased, but our bodies are suffering under the constant increase and decrease of blood sugar levels.

2. Nutrient density has decreased even though our calorie intake has spiked. Processed foods are rich in calories but poor in

nutritional value, and they don't satisfy your hunger as whole foods do. Processed foods don't contain nutrients responsible for signaling to our brains that we're full and nourished; thus, our bodies keep sending hunger signals to the brain. This is why it's so easy to overconsume processed foods.

3. Healthy fats have been replaced with vegetable oil and margarine. When consumed excessively, this can create or promote inflammation in the body. "Vegetable oils" refer to sunflower oil, safflower oil, canola oil, and corn oil. Coconut and olive oils are highly nutritious and should be opted for instead of the former. Vegetable oils are high in trans fats, increasing the risk of diabetes, heart disease, and obesity. Frequent consumption of omega-6s can interfere with the balance of omega-3s and -6s of the cells, which can result in a number of problems.

Health is not just defined as the absence of disease in humans. It's about mental, social, and physical well-being. When you're healthy, you tackle your daily tasks effectively. Healthy people are more productive at work and have the energy to exercise and the mental capacity to cope better with stressful situations. The keto diet is a great way to work your way to a state of complete health.

Some Things Worth Considering

Even though the ketogenic diet has many benefits to offer, it's not for everyone. Like any other diet, there are a few exceptions where people can't take the risk of following a ketogenic diet without consulting a medical practitioner. Before you get on board, there are some steps to take to prepare yourself.

Get to Know What Foods to Eat and What to Avoid

There's more to the keto diet than just avoiding sugar and foods that you may think do not contain a lot of carbs. A quick peek at the nutritional value of packaged foods simply won't do. Try to steer clear of any packaged foods, and fill your shopping cart with the following delicious whole foods to kickstart your keto diet:

1. Seafood. Sardines, mackerel, salmon, and other fish are high in omega-3 fatty acids, and they've been shown to lower insulin levels in people who are overweight or obese. Some shellfish may contain more carbs than others. Opt for clams, mussels, octopus, squid, and oysters. These contain three to four grams of carbohydrates per 3.5-ounce serving.
2. Cheese. This may be the best thing for keto followers about the diet; the fact that you're allowed to eat and enjoy cheese! A study showed that eating cheese regularly may help you build muscle mass and strength. The following cheeses are allowed on the keto diet:
    - Goat cheese
    - Feta
    - Halloumi
    - Cottage cheese
    - Blue cheese
    - Brie
    - Camembert
    - Chevre
    - Cheddar
    - Mozzarella
    - Pepper Jack
    - String cheese
    - Swiss
    - Romano
    - Muenster

- Manchego
- Limburger
- Mascarpone
- Cream cheese
- Cottage cheese
- Provolone

3. Avocado. They're packed with minerals and potassium, plus they're super healthy! One half of a medium-sized avocado contains nine grams of carbs; their net carb count is only two grams because seven of these carbs are fiber. A higher potassium intake might make it easier for you to make the transition from your normal diet to the keto diet. Avocados have also been shown to lower bad cholesterol (LDL) levels and improve triglyceride levels.
4. Eggs. They're healthy and versatile, and one large egg contains one gram of carbs and six grams of protein. It is truly the ideal food for the ketogenic diet. A study found that eggs cause hormones that are responsible for feeling full to be released. Even though they're high in cholesterol, they have been shown to reduce the risk of heart disease. Most of the egg's nutrients are found in the yolk, so enjoy the whole egg!
5. Meat and poultry. Meat-eaters, this one's for you! Poultry and fresh meat contain no carbs, and they're an excellent source of protein (don't eat too much of them, though) that will aid in preserving muscle mass when following a low-carb diet. Opt for grass-fed meat if possible because it's higher in omega-3 fatty acids and antioxidants than grain-fed meat.
6. Low-carb veggies. Consuming high-carb vegetables such as potatoes, yams, or beets may put you over your carb limit for the day. There are many low-carb vegetables that you can eat that are high in fiber and vitamins. Low-carb veggies such as cauliflower and zucchini can be a great substitution for high-carb foods. For example, you can make cauliflower rice or

mash and zucchini noodles. The following vegetables are keto-friendly:
- Green beans
- Cucumbers
- Cauliflower
- Kale
- Olives
- Lettuce
- Asparagus
- Broccoli
- Cabbage
- Eggplant
- Spinach
- Tomatoes
- Peppers (green are best)
- Zucchini
- Avocado (even though it's technically a fruit)
- Brussel sprouts
- Celery

7. Plain Greek yogurt. It promotes the feeling of being full and helps to decrease appetite. It should be taken in moderation as it contains some carbs. One cup of Greek yogurt contains nine grams of protein and only four grams of carbs.
8. Olive oil. The ideal base for salad dressings and healthy mayonnaise! It's a pure source of fat, so it contains no carbs. It's high in antioxidants such as phenol, which has been shown to improve artery function and decrease the risk of heart disease.
9. Coconut oil. It's been used to increase ketones in people with nervous system disorders and Alzheimer's disease. This is because it contains medium-chain triglycerides (MCTs); the liver takes them up directly and converts these MCTs into ketones. It has been suggested that MCTs can sustain your level

of ketosis. Coconut oil may reduce belly fat in adults who are obese; one study showed men eating two tablespoons of coconut oil per day lost an average of one inch without making any dietary changes.

10. Nuts and seeds. They're high in fiber and fat, and they don't contain a lot of calories. Nuts and seeds can help you absorb fewer calories. The regular consumption of nuts has been linked to a reduced risk of certain cancers, depression, heart disease, and other chronic diseases. The carb count varies for different types of nuts and seeds. Here are the carb counts for one ounce of the popular nuts and seeds:
    - Brazil nuts contain 1g net carbs and a total of 3g carbs.
    - Pistachios contain 5g net carbs and a total of 8g carbs.
    - Walnuts contain 2g net carbs and a total of 4g carbs.
    - Macadamia nuts contain 2g net carbs and a total of 4g carbs.
    - Almonds contain 2g net carbs and a total of 6g carbs.
    - Cashew nuts contain 8g net carbs and a total of 9g carbs.
    - Flaxseeds contain 0g net carbs and a total of 8g carbs.
    - Sesame seeds contain 3g of net carbs and a total of 7g carbs.
    - Chia seeds contain 1g net carbs and a total of 12g carbs.
    - Pumpkin seeds contain 3g net carbs and a total of 5g carbs.
11. Cream and butter. Containing only trace amounts of carbohydrates, these are the ideal additions to the keto diet. Cream and butter are high in saturated fats, which have no link to heart disease for most people. They are rich in conjugated linoleic acid that may promote weight loss. Studies have shown that moderate consumption of butter and cream has beneficial effects on heart health.

12. Berries. They're the exception on a keto diet as most fruits are too high in carbohydrates to be included in this diet. They're high in fiber and contain few carbs, and they're packed with antioxidants that have been shown to reduce inflammation and protect us from diseases. Let's look at the carb counts for 3.5 ounces of the following berries:
    - Blackberries have a total of 16g carbs but contain a net amount of 11g carbs.
    - Strawberries have a total of 9g of carbs but contain a net amount of 6g carbs.
    - Raspberries have a total of 12g carbs but contain a net amount of 6g carbs.
    - Blueberries have a total of 12g carbs but a net amount of 9g of carbs.
13. Dark chocolate and cocoa powder. Dark chocolate may lower blood pressure and keep your arteries healthy because it contains flavonoids (a type of plant nutrient). There are only three grams net carbs in one ounce of dark (100% cocoa), unsweetened chocolate. Much to the surprise of chocolate lovers, it may be included in the keto diet. The trick is to choose chocolate that has at least 70% cocoa solids. It's important to keep in mind that moderation is key!

The hardest thing about starting the keto diet is old habits. It's not easy giving up high-carb food; we're so familiar with it, and until now, we probably haven't thought of the effects that some of these foods may have on our bodies.

You'll want to avoid the following foods due to their carb counts or the amount of sugar they contain:

1. Bread and grains. Even though these are a staple food for many, they should be avoided on the keto diet because they contain high carb counts. If you feel that it would be

impossible to give up bread, you can make your own low-carb loaves at home!
2. Fruit. Except for berries, most fruits are high in carbs, making them unsuitable for the keto diet. For example, a small apple contains 21 grams of carbs, four of which come from fiber.
3. Beer. It's well known that beer is high in carbs. You can still enjoy a drink on the keto diet, though. Hard liquor has zero grams of carbs, and dry red wine has a low carb count. Studies have shown that liquid carbs may increase your risk of weight gain more than carbs from solid foods.
4. Juice. Did you know that apple juice contains more carbs than soda? It seems almost impossible, but 12 ounces of apple juice contains 48 grams of carbs. A can of soda contains 39 grams of carbs. Drinking juice can promote the feeling of hunger since the brain may not process these liquid carbs the same way as solid carbs. Fruit juice is one of the worst drinks you can consume when following a low-carb diet.
5. Beans and legumes. These may be taken in moderation depending on your tolerance and daily carb limit. They do contain a high carb count, but they're rich in fiber and contribute to heart health and the reduction of inflammation. Small portions are allowed, so here are the carb counts for one cup of the following beans and legumes:
    - Black beans contain a total of 41g carbs, of which 15 are fiber.
    - Chickpeas contain a total of 45g carbs, of which 12 are fiber.
    - Lentils contain a total of 40g carbs, of which 16 are fiber.
    - Pinto beans contain a total of 45g carbs, of which 15 are fiber.
    - Kidney beans contain a total of 40g carbs, of which 13 are fiber.

- Peas contain a total of 25g carbs, of which 9 are fiber.

For vegans and vegetarians, try to consume a third of a cup instead of one whole cup to lower your carb intake. Beans and legumes are very nutritious, so smaller portions should suffice!

6. Honey or any form of sugar. Natural sugar can have as many carbs as refined sugar, and it contains no nutritional value. It's best to steer clear of it completely. To sweeten food or beverages, opt for a healthy sweetener instead.
7. Gluten-free baked goods. They may contain a higher carb count than glutenous foods. This is because the flour used to bake these goods is made from grains and starches, which can spike your blood sugar levels. Stick to making your own bread with coconut or almond flour rather than consuming processed gluten-free food.
8. Milk. It contains too many carbs to be included in your keto diet. Instead, opt for cream, unsweetened coconut milk, or almond milk.
9. Any processed snack foods. Even whole wheat crackers are a no-go on the keto diet. Snacks like chips and crackers are high in carbs, and it's best to avoid them completely.

Take Note of the Downsides of a Keto diet

- Athletic impediments. Even though the keto diet boosts your energy after a few weeks, research on the long-term effects that a ketogenic diet might have on people who train intensively is lacking. Carbs are necessary to produce insulin that plays a role in driving protein into muscles faster. Insulin is also responsible for building up glycogen stores for longer training sessions such as hiking or running.
- Keto "flu." The keto diet is extreme, so the transition won't necessarily be easy. You might experience some symptoms

such as brain fog, nausea, headaches, and fatigue. Some beginners have also reported bad breath, frequent urination, and excessive sweating. This is because the keto diet influences your electrolyte balance, and the acetone must seep out somehow, right? Luckily, these symptoms are temporary and will disappear after the first seven to ten days. The secret to minimizing your risk of the keto flu and constipation is the consumption of fluids. Be sure to drink enough water and other keto-friendly drinks. You can also start by following a regular low-carb diet to teach your body to burn fat without eliminating carbs.

- Constipation. When starting, you will experience some bowel issues. This is mainly because whole grains and fruit are cut out of your diet. The good news is that you can consume fiber-rich vegetables or nuts and seeds to prevent constipation!

You Might Experience Some Nutrient Deficiencies

As with any restrictive diet, cutting out certain foods may result in you missing out on some important nutrients. Some of the big ones are:

- Sodium. When your carb intake is limited, insulin production declines and your kidneys absorb less sodium and excrete more waste. To prevent symptoms of grumpiness, fatigue, and dizziness, season your food with sea salt.
- Potassium. The food list on the keto diet is limited, and the absence of some fruit that provides a dose of potassium may cause constipation accompanied by stomach cramps. Make sure that you eat enough spinach, tomatoes, and avocado to prevent a potassium deficiency.
- Vitamin C. Your vegetable intake should compensate for the vitamin C you're missing out on by cutting most fruit from

your diet. Make sure you eat enough broccoli, cabbage, and cauliflower to prevent a vitamin C deficiency.
- The prevention of some nutrient deficiencies involves a balance of substitutions that contain the same nutrients. The best way to start is slowly. Be patient with yourself, and start by making small changes to your diet. For example, you can start by cutting starch and sugary snacks and drinks from your diet. After that, kick it up a notch by cutting starchy vegetables and processed food. Starting small can increase your chances of successfully sticking to this diet.

The secret to minimizing your risk of the keto flu and constipation is the consumption of fluids. Be sure to drink enough water and other keto-friendly drinks. You can also start by following a regular low-carb diet.

Have a long-term plan to maintain your weight loss since the keto diet is not a long-term solution. Studies recommend not following the diet for more than 12 weeks at a time. So be sure to have an eating plan ready when you're taking a break from keto.

Keto Tips and Tricks

The keto diet doesn't have to be a challenging transition! There are many ways to make it easy for yourself, even in social settings! The results, symptoms, and effects of the keto diet will differ from person to person. There are some groups that should steer clear of it completely or consider asking for advice from a medical professional.

Who Should Steer Clear of the Keto Diet?

As mentioned before, the keto diet is not for everyone. It's important that you consult a medical practitioner to give you advice on how to start and to help you stay on the right track without putting your health in danger. An example of some groups that shouldn't try the keto diet includes:

- Healthy children. A variety of nutrients are important for the healthy growth and development of kids. The keto diet is too extreme for healthy children to follow. More importantly, childhood is no time for dieting.
- Pregnant and breastfeeding women. Since research suggests metabolic changes occur during ketosis, the risk of stunted fetal growth increases should pregnant women follow a ketogenic diet. Pregnant women should not risk undernourishing themselves as extreme weight loss can have a negative impact on the milk supply.
- People with kidney issues. The shift in sodium, potassium, and fluid balance can have a negative impact on people with kidney stones.
- Gastrointestinal surgery patients, people with pancreatic issues, and people with gallbladder problems. As people who have had gastrointestinal surgery have limited digestive abilities, it's best that they steer clear of the keto diet. Fat is particularly difficult to digest, which is why it's not recommended for these groups.
- People with a history of eating disorders. The extremity of the keto diet may trigger disordered eating thoughts.

To Get Started

The transition from your modern-day diet to the keto diet can be challenging, so start by applying these simple changes:

- Plan your meals for the week in advance. Before the start of a new week, prepare snacks or make your mayonnaise or salad dressing and store them for the week ahead. This can save you some time and help you stick to your diet.

- Familiarize yourself with some delicious keto recipes, and start teaching yourself how to cook if you can't. There are many delicious keto recipes you have to try!
- Learn to look at the nutritional information of foods. Check for grams of fat, carbs, and fiber to try to incorporate some of your favorite foods into your diet.
- Start looking into frozen keto meals. This is not ideal, but if you lack the time and cooking skills, it's a viable option. Alternatively, there are a lot of food delivery services that offer keto-friendly options.
- Consider packing your own food when visiting family and friends. This is the best way to stick to your diet and keep your cravings under control when attending social gatherings.
- When visiting a restaurant, opt for egg-based meals such as omelets or bacon and eggs (without toast or fries). Most restaurants offer fish dishes, so swap out the high-carb foods for veggies. You can even enjoy a bun-less burger and top it with avocado, eggs, or bacon.

Being social doesn't have to be difficult when following a ketogenic diet!

As a Beginner, Consider Other Methods of the Keto Diet

There are several different keto diets available for you to choose from! Some of these include:

- Standard Keto Diet (SKD). The most extreme keto diet is the SKD. It's a very low-carb, high-fat, and moderate-protein diet. It calls for 70% fat, 20% protein, and 10% carbs.
- High-Protein Keto Diet. This diet is almost like the SKD, but it includes more protein. So, the ratio is 60% fat, 5% carbs, and 35% protein.

- Targeted Keto Diet (TKD). TKD allows you to add more carbs around workouts.
- Cyclical Keto Diet (CKD). This diet allows for a higher carb intake on certain days. For example, five ketogenic days and two high-carb days.

There aren't many studies on the TKD or the CKD, but they are primarily used by athletes and are a more advanced method of following a ketogenic diet.

11 Frequently Asked Questions

Some of the most common questions about the ketogenic diet are:

1. Will I ever eat carbs again?

While on the diet, no. But after two or three months, allow yourself some carbs on special occasions. Just be sure to return to the keto diet immediately after.

2. How much protein can I eat?

Try not to exceed 35%. Protein should be moderate on the ketogenic diet since a high protein intake can spike insulin levels and, as a result, reduce ketone production.

3. Won't I lose muscle?

Protein intake and ketones can prevent the loss of muscle, but the risk of some muscle loss comes with every diet. To minimize muscle loss, you can lift weights or do some strength training exercises.

4. Can I build muscle on a ketogenic diet?

It might not work as well as on a moderate carb diet, but it is possible. As mentioned previously, there are other keto diet methods that can be considered.

   5. Why does my urine smell fruity?

The fruity smell is due to the process of waste excretion caused by ketosis. It is nothing to be alarmed about.

   6. Won't I constantly feel tired and weak?

Fatigue and weakness will only last a couple of days. If this is not the case, you might not be utilizing fats and ketones efficiently. A supplement may help for this, such as ketones or MCT oil.

   7. Why does my breath smell?

Bad breath is a common side effect of the ketogenic diet. It's due to the excretion of acetone during ketosis. You can chew on a piece of sugar-free gum or sip on naturally flavored water to combat this; it will subside after a few days.

   8. Is ketosis dangerous?

People seem to confuse ketosis with ketoacidosis. Ketoacidosis is dangerous, but ketosis on the keto diet is usually fine for healthy people.

   9. I have diarrhea and digestion issues. What should I do?

This is a common side effect of the keto diet and will pass after three to four weeks. Should the problem persist, opt for fiber-rich veggies.

   10. How much weight will I lose?

It totally depends on you. You'll start losing weight within the first few days of being on the keto diet, but adding exercise to your routine can speed up the process.

   11. What supplements should I take?

There's a good chance that you'll get a good balance of nutrients when following the keto diet. However, if you don't feel "right" after you've started with this diet, there are a few supplements that you can consider taking:

- Minerals. Since there will be a shift in the balance of minerals, this is a useful supplement you can use.
- Exogenous ketones. These can help raise the body's ketone levels.
- Whey protein powder. Increase your daily protein intake by adding half a scoop to your yogurt.
- Caffeine. It has been shown to have fat-burning, increased performance, and energy-boosting abilities.
- Creatine. If you are combining the keto diet with exercise, creatine can have many benefits for your health and performance.
- MCT oil. You can add a few drops to your drinks or yogurt for an energy boost. It also aids in increased ketone levels.

If you follow the keto diet to a T, you shouldn't have trouble getting all of the important nutrients that your body needs. A lot of the foods that are allowed on the keto diet can provide sufficient nutrients and minerals. Even though there will be some side effects after you've started with the keto diet, they won't last long. If you can push through them, you'll start reaping the benefits within the first few weeks.

If you plan on easing yourself into the carb-cutting requirements of the keto diet, there is another way to get a jumpstart on ketone production. It's mostly safe, effective, and a great practice run for maintaining your newly motivated healthy lifestyle!

Chapter 3:

Intermittent Fasting

Intermittent fasting is a weight-loss method that involves restricting calories by fasting for the majority of the day and the normal consumption of food within a specific time. There are various fasting routines such as:

- The 16/8 method. It involves eating within a time frame of 8 hours and then abstaining from food for 16 hours. You can skip breakfast, start eating at 12 p.m., and have your last meal by 8 p.m. This is one of the most popular fasting routines since many people already skip breakfast. It is also considered the easiest method of fasting since you don't eat anything after dinner until noon the next day.
- The 5:2 diet (also known as the Fast Diet). This method of fasting was popularized by British journalist Michael Mosley. It involves normal food consumption for five days a week and restricting calories for two nonconsecutive days of the week. Women are recommended to consume no more than 500 calories on restricting days, whereas men should consume only 600 calories.
- The eat-stop-eat method. This method involves fasting for 24 hours at least once or twice per week. You'll eat normally for four or five days a week and fast for 24 hours every other day. For example, on Monday, you'll eat your last meal at 6 p.m. and only have dinner again at 6 p.m. the next day. It's important that you stay hydrated during the fasting period, but no solid foods are allowed. Stick to water, coffee, and zero-calorie drinks during your fasting period. If you choose to do this

method to lose weight, it's important that you eat the same amount of food that you normally would during the eating period. This is a little more advanced method of fasting, so start with an easier method before trying this one.
- Alternate-day fasting. This method involves fasting every other day. It's not necessarily a method that calls for 24 hours of fasting since you can choose to restrict your calories every other day if you're a beginner. A full fast every other day is rather extreme for beginners, so restrict your calories at first and work your way to a full fast.
- Spontaneous meal skipping. This method is the easiest way of practicing intermittent fasting and a great way to start! It involves skipping a meal when you're simply not hungry or don't have the time to eat. Just make sure that you eat healthy meals when you do eat.
- The warrior diet. It involves eating small amounts of raw fruits and vegetables during the day and having one large meal for dinner. You'll fast all day by restricting calories and eat at night within a four-hour eating window.

To many, this might seem strange. We have been told that breakfast is the most important meal of the day and that we should eat three or more times per day. Fasting has been around for a long time; it's not a new fad or crazy marketing scheme. It's been practiced by religious groups, and medical practitioners have recommended it for various health benefits for centuries.

The Benefits of Intermittent Fasting

Intermittent fasting is a great way to lose fat! The first step to understanding how intermittent fasting can lead to fat loss is to know the difference between the fed state and the fasted state. After a meal, your body is in the fed state. This simply means that your body is digesting and absorbing food; it starts when you eat and lasts for approximately three to five hours. In the fed state, you're not burning fat due to elevated insulin levels.

After the three- to five-hour time span, your body stops processing and absorbing food. This is known as the postabsorptive state, and it lasts for eight to twelve hours after your last meal, after which you've entered the fasted state. In the fasted state, your insulin levels are low, making it easier for your body to burn fat. This state allows your body to burn fat that has been inaccessible instead of continuously processing and absorbing food. The problem with eating too often is that we don't allow our bodies to enter the fasted state.

While fat loss is great, it isn't the only benefit of intermittent fasting.

It Can Alter the Function of Genes, Hormones, and Cells

When you don't eat, your body initiates changes in hormone levels and cellular repair to make stored fat easily accessible. Numerous changes occur such as:

- Insulin levels decrease significantly, which initiates fat burning.
- Important cellular repair processes are induced to remove waste material from cells.
- Human growth hormone levels increase. This can facilitate muscle gain and help you burn fat.
- Several changes occur in genes and molecules relating to longevity and protection from disease.

Many of the intermittent fasting benefits are related to these changes.

It Can Lower Your Risk of Type 2 Diabetes

Intermittent fasting has been linked to lowering blood sugar levels, therefore decreasing insulin resistance. A study in humans found that intermittent fasting reduced fasting blood sugar levels by 3-6%, and fasting insulin was reduced by 20-31%. A study in diabetic rats also showed that intermittent fasting protected them from kidney disease, which is one of the most severe complications of diabetes. It goes to show that intermittent fasting can protect people who are at risk of developing type 2 diabetes. There may be some differences depending on gender, as one study showed that the blood sugar control in women worsened after 22 days of intermittent fasting.

It Can Reduce Inflammation and Oxidative Stress in the Body

Oxidative stress involves unstable molecules (free radicals) damaging important molecules such as DNA or protein. Oxidative stress causes aging and many chronic diseases. Luckily, intermittent fasting has been shown to reduce oxidative stress in the body. Additionally, intermittent fasting has been shown to reduce inflammation, which is another key driver of various chronic diseases.

It May Be Beneficial for Heart Health

A lot of evidence on the benefits of intermittent fasting on heart health is based on animal studies. But it has proved to reduce numerous risk factors such as high blood pressure, inflammatory markers, LDL cholesterol, triglycerides, and blood sugar levels. Heart disease is currently one of the world's biggest killers, and health markers are associated with an increased or decreased risk of heart disease. Further studies in humans are needed before any recommendations can be made, so it's important to consult a medical practitioner before you decide to try intermittent fasting.

It May Extend Your Lifespan

Studies in rats showed significant effects on their lifespan. These studies showed that fasting every other day extended the rats' lifespans by up to 83%. Since there are many known benefits to the effect that intermittent fasting has on metabolism and many health markers, it makes sense that it could help us live longer and healthier. Further studies in humans need to be done before this can be proven.

So, what links intermittent fasting and the keto diet? Both initiate the process of ketosis, which is responsible for all of the possible health benefits. You could jumpstart the production of ketones by trying a fasting method for a few days before you start the keto diet. Intermittent fasting is a pattern of eating instead of a diet. Mainly, people try it to lose fat. It is one of the simplest strategies to lose weight because it doesn't require a lot of behavioral changes. Intermittent fasting is a great way to maintain your weight after the keto diet and to keep your eating habits under control.

Combining the Keto Diet With Intermittent Fasting

Even though fasting is not necessary to reach ketosis when following a ketogenic diet, it can speed up the process. Combining the two is safe for healthy people, and it will help you reach your weight-loss goals faster. Both can produce higher energy levels and lead to a dramatic loss of fat without losing muscle mass. In one study involving 34 resistance-trained men, those who practiced the 16/8 intermittent fasting method lost almost 14% more body fat than those who stuck to normal eating patterns over eight weeks.

Since intermittent fasting preserves muscle mass while losing weight, it can be helpful for people who are looking to drop body fat and improve athletic performance. For anyone who struggles to experience ketosis on the keto diet, intermittent fasting can help jumpstart the process. While the combining method may work for some, it's important to note that it won't work the same for everyone. It's not necessary to do both, but there's nothing wrong with trying to experiment a little.

Some may find that practicing intermittent fasting is too difficult while following the ketogenic diet; it can trigger people to overeat on non-fasting days and cause irritability and fatigue. But it is a good way to teach yourself that you'll survive without food for a couple of hours.

Chapter 4:

A 14-Day Meal Plan With Recipes for Meat Eaters

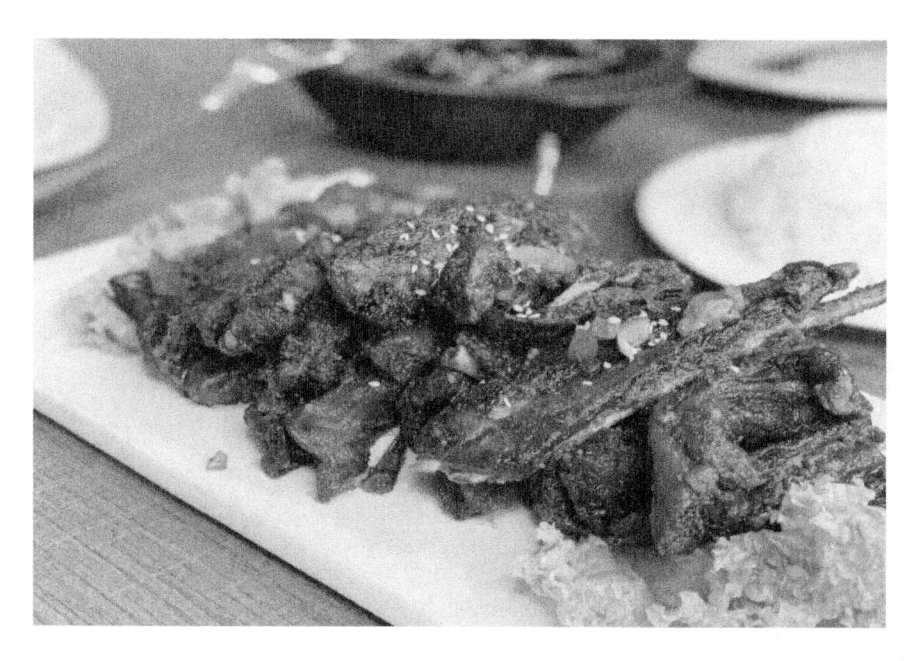

The meal plan you're about to read can be easily adjusted to fit your needs and time. To save cooking time:

- Keep your pantry stocked with olive oil, avocado, eggs, and bacon for quick and easy high-fat, low-carb breakfasts, lunches, or healthy snacks.
- Have enough cooked meat stored in the fridge. You can slow-cook or prepare roast meat every Sunday to have some cooking

meats during the week. It's as easy as adding these meats to soup, stir-fry, or salads.
- Make large enough portions of keto casserole dishes or stews each week. You can eat multiple dinners or lunches from these dishes.

For the first week, try to cook meals that you already know and enjoy, made keto. This will make the transition a little easier and prevent you from feeling unsatisfied or like you're missing out. You aren't obligated to stick to this meal plan; have breakfast for lunch if you don't normally eat breakfast, or have lunch for dinner if you're not in the mood to eat anything too heavy. This is just an idea of what a keto meal plan can look like. As long as you're not consuming sugar or starch, you'll do just fine! These meals are so delicious you won't feel like you're missing out on anything. Breakfast is always optional if you're trying to incorporate intermittent fasting into your routine. The keto coffees can be consumed during your fasting period as they're super low in carbs. These coffees will not break your fast.

Day 1

Breakfast (Optional): Traditional Keto Coffee

Time: 2 minutes

Makes: 1 cup

Prep Time: 2 minutes

Nutritional Value (per serving):

Net carbs	*0g*
Fat	*17g*
Protein	*0g*
Calories	*143*

Ingredients:
- 1 cup black coffee
- ½ tsp MCT oil (add more once you know you can handle it)
- 1 tbsp ghee

Directions:
1. Using a milk frother or a blender, add the ingredients and mix well until foam forms.

Lunch: Creamy Salmon and Zucchini Pasta

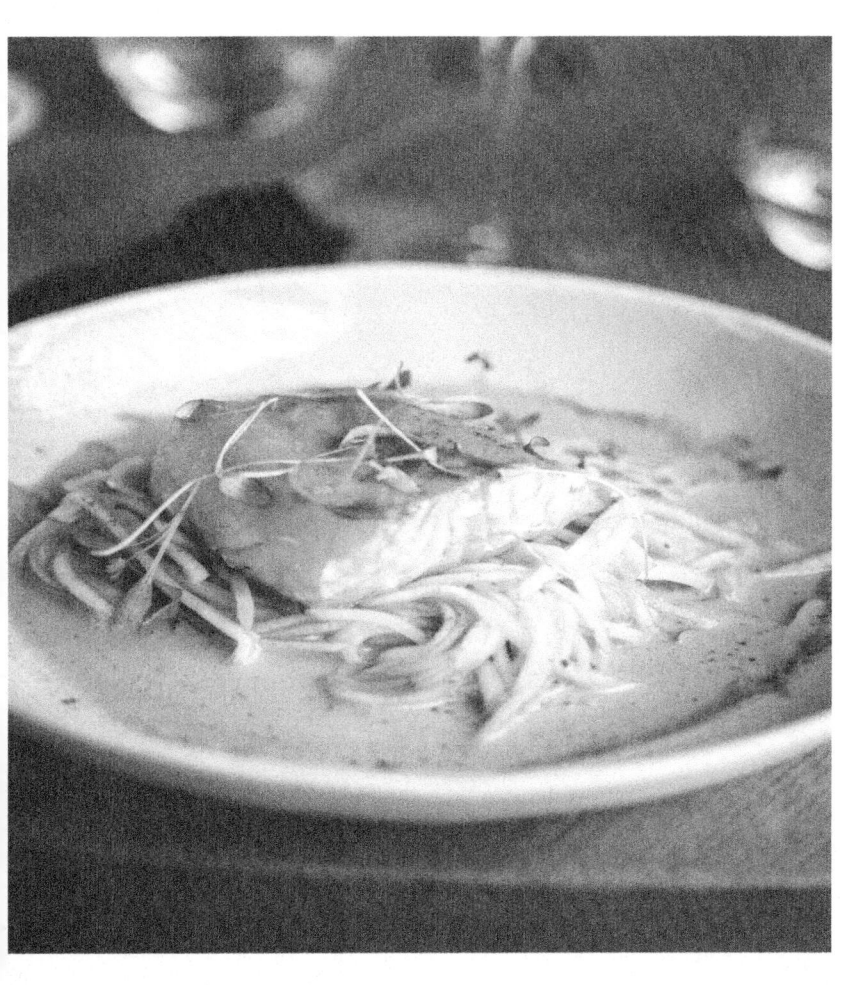

Time: 10 minutes

Makes: 2 servings

Prep Time: 5 minutes

Cook Time: 5 minutes

Nutritional Value (per serving):

Net carbs	*3g*
Fat	*42g*
Protein	*21g*
Calories	*470*

Ingredients:

- 2 tbsp coconut oil to cook with
- 8 oz diced smoked salmon
- 2 zucchinis, make strands with a potato peeler so that they resemble noodles
- ¼ cup mayonnaise

Directions:

1. Using a frying pan, melt the coconut oil on medium-high heat before adding the salmon cubes. Fry the cubes for approximately 2 minutes or until they turn a honey-brown color.
2. Mix your zucchini noodles with the salmon cubes and fry everything for approximately 2 minutes before stirring in the mayonnaise.
3. Divide your "pasta" in half, serve, and enjoy!

Dinner: One-Pot Chicken and Broccoli Delight

Time: 1 hour and 15 minutes

Makes: 6 servings

Prep Time: 15 minutes

Cook Time: 1 hour

Nutritional Value (per serving):

Net carbs	9g
Fat	29g
Protein	20g
Calories	389

Ingredients:
- 2 diced chicken breasts
- 1 head cauliflower florets
- 1 head broccoli florets
- ½ medium onion, diced
- 3 tbsp chopped fresh thyme
- 2 tbsp chopped fresh parsley
- 1 tbsp garlic powder
- 4 sliced white button mushrooms
- 1 cup coconut cream
- 2 tbsp ghee, melted
- 4 tbsp coconut oil to cook the chicken
- Salt and pepper to taste

Directions:

1. While your oven is preheating to 350°F, cook the salt-and-pepper seasoned chicken in a pan with coconut oil.
2. In a baking pan, add ghee and then the rest of the ingredients before popping the pan into the oven and allowing it to cook uncovered for 1 hour.
3. Serve, and store the rest in an airtight container in the fridge.

Day 2

Breakfast (Optional): Creamy Coconut Coffee

Time: 2 minutes

Makes: 1 cup

Prep Time: 2 minutes

Nutritional Value (per serving):

Net carbs	*0g*
Fat	*21g*
Protein	*0g*
Calories	*179*

Ingredients:

- 1 cup black coffee
- ½ tbsp coconut oil
- 1 tbsp ghee

Directions:

1. Using a blender or a milk frother, combine and mix the ingredients until foamy.

Lunch: Spanish Omelet

Time: 40 minutes

Makes: 4 servings

Cook Time: 30 minutes

Prep Time: 10 minutes

Nutritional Value (per serving):

Net carbs	*10g*
Fat	*22g*
Protein	*14g*
Calories	*286*

Ingredients:

- 2 tbsp olive oil for cooking
- 2 diced medium bell peppers
- 1 diced medium onion

- ½ head chopped cauliflower
- 8 medium-sized eggs, whisked
- ¼ cup coconut cream
- 4 tbsp chopped parsley
- Salt and pepper to taste

Directions:

1. While the oven is preheating to 350°F, boil the cauliflower in water for 2 minutes and strain it. Set it aside.
2. In a pan, fry the onions and bell peppers in olive oil and season with salt and pepper to taste.
3. In a bowl, combine the eggs, parsley, strained cauliflower, and fried bell pepper and onion, and add the coconut cream.
4. Pour the combination into a square baking tray and lay out the vegetables evenly before placing them in the oven to cook for approximately 20 minutes.
5. Cut your omelet in 4 quarters, serve, and store the remainder of this dish in an airtight container in the fridge.

Dinner: Sautéed Vegetables With Lemony Garlic Salmon

Time: 30 minutes

Makes: 2 servings

Prep Time: 10 minutes

Cook Time: 20 minutes

Nutritional Value (per serving):

Net carbs	11g
Fat	51g
Protein	43g
Calories	680

Ingredients:

- 10 spears asparagus, chopped
- 1 leek, chopped
- 2 tsp ginger powder
- Avocado or olive oil for frying
- 2 tbsp lemon juice
- Salt to taste
- 2 salmon fillets (keep the skin on)
- 1 tbsp ghee
- 4 garlic cloves, minced
- Lemon slice for serving

Directions:

1. Season your salmon fillets with ghee, 1 tbsp of lemon juice, minced garlic, and a sprinkle of salt, and wrap them in aluminum foil or parchment paper while the oven is preheating to 400°F.
2. Cook the wrapped salmon in the oven. After 10 minutes, remove the foil or the parchment paper package from the oven, partially unwrap the salmon and place it back into the oven to cook for another 10 minutes.
3. While you wait for your salmon to finish cooking, fry the chopped asparagus and leek in olive oil for 10 minutes before

mixing in ginger powder, 1 tbsp of lemon juice, and salt, and fry for 1 more minute.
4. Serve by dividing the vegetables in half, place half of the vegetables on a plate and top them with your delicious salmon fillet.

Day 3

Breakfast (Optional): Bacon and Chicken Sausages

Time: 30 minutes

Makes: 12 sausages

Prep Time: 10 minutes

Cook Time: 20 minutes

Nutritional Value (per serving):

Net carbs	3g
Fat	21g
Protein	40g
Calories	370

Ingredients:
- 1 lb ground chicken
- 2 slices cooked bacon, chopped
- 1 egg, whisked

- 2 tbsp Italian seasoning
- 2 tsp garlic powder
- 1 tsp onion powder
- Salt and pepper to taste

Directions:
1. While the oven is preheating to 425°F, run all the ingredients through a food processor.
2. Place foil in a baking pan before placing 12 thinly formed (about ½ inch) patties on the foil.
3. Pop the baking pan in the oven for approximately 20 minutes. The internal temperature of the patties placed in the middle of the pan should be 170°F. You can also pan-fry them instead of baking them in the oven.
4. You can store them in the fridge and reheat them in the microwave for a quick and easy breakfast.

Lunch: Baked Egg in Avocado (a keto favorite)

Time: 17 minutes

Serving Size: 2 servings

Prep Time: 5 minutes

Cook Time: 12 minutes

Nutritional Value (per serving):

Net carbs	*9g*
Fat	*23g*
Protein	*3g*
Calories	*250*

Ingredients:

- 1 avocado
- 2 egg yolks
- 2 tsp olive oil or coconut oil
- Salt and pepper to taste
- Smoked paprika to taste

Directions:

1. Slice the avocado in half and remove the stone, wrapping the outsides of the avocado in aluminum foil (keep the peel on for easy serving) while the oven is preheating to 400°F.
2. Break two eggs open carefully and separate the yolks. Put the egg yolks in the avocado halves and drizzle 1 tsp of olive or coconut oil over the egg yolks.
3. Cook them in the oven for 12 minutes or until the egg yolks are soft but not too runny.
4. Season with salt, pepper, and smoked paprika to taste and enjoy!

Dinner: Potato less Cottage Pie

Time: 1 hour

Makes: 4 servings

Prep Time: 15 minutes

Cook Time: 45 minutes

Nutritional Value (per serving):

Net carbs	*8g*
Fat	*57g*
Protein	*32g*
Calories	*684*

Ingredients:
- 1 head worth of cauliflower florets
- 2 tbsp melted ghee
- ¼ cup avocado oil to cook beef
- 1 medium finely chopped onion
- 2 carrots, grated
- 1 ½ lbs ground beef
- 2 tbsp Italian seasoning
- 2 tbsp chopped fresh parsley
- Salt and pepper to taste
- A handful of crushed nuts and seeds

Directions:

1. Boil or steam the cauliflower florets for approximately 5 to 10 minutes (depending on the size of the florets) or until soft while the oven is preheating to 350°F.
2. Strain the cooked cauliflower well and add them to a blender along with ghee and salt to taste. Blend the mixture until smooth or until it resembles mashed potatoes. Place it to the side and grease an oven tray.
3. In a pan, fry onions in avocado oil until they develop a translucent color before placing the ground beef and carrots in the pan. Fry for about 10 minutes, then season with Italian seasoning and parsley. Sprinkle it with salt and pepper to taste.
4. Spread the beef combination in the bottom of your greased baking tray.
5. Spread the mashed cauliflower over the beef mixture and pop it in the oven for 30 minutes or until golden brown.
6. Let your delicious dish cool down before serving, divide it into 4 portions, and enjoy! You can store the remainder of your keto cottage pie in the fridge.

Day 4

Breakfast: Easy Keto Frittatas

Time: 40 minutes

Makes: 12 muffins

Prep Time: 10 minutes

Cook Time: 30 minutes

Nutritional Value (per serving):

Net carbs	3g
Fat	41g
Protein	19g
Calories	460

Ingredients:

- 1 cup chopped asparagus
- 4 slices diced bacon
- 2 tbsp chopped onion
- 8 eggs, whisked
- ½ cup coconut milk
- Salt and pepper to taste

Directions:

1. While the oven is preheating to 350°F, fry the bacon in a pan.
2. In a bowl, combine the eggs, coconut milk, cooked bacon, and chopped vegetables.
3. Make 12 mini quiches by pouring the combination into a silicone muffin pan, and then pop them in the oven for 25 to 30 minutes.
4. You now have a yummy breakfast or lunch that's sure to make you feel full for longer!

Lunch: Chicken and Zucchini Noodle Soup

Time: 30 minutes

Makes: 2 bowls

Prep Time: 15 minutes

Cook Time: 15 minutes

Nutritional Value (per serving):

Net carbs	6g
Fat	16g
Protein	34g
Calories	310

Ingredients:
- 3 cups chicken broth
- 1 chopped chicken breast
- 2 tbsp avocado oil
- 1 stalk chopped celery
- 1 finely chopped green onion
- ¼ cup chopped cilantro
- 1 peeled zucchini
- Salt to taste

Directions:
1. Fry the diced chicken in avocado oil until cooked in a pan. Pour in chicken broth and allow it to boil on medium to low heat.

2. Introduce the chopped celery and green onion to the chicken mixture.
3. Make zucchini noodles with a potato peeler and mix your noodles along with the chopped cilantro into the chicken and vegetable mixture.
4. Boil it for a few more minutes, sprinkle with salt to taste, and serve.

Dinner: Sesame Beef Teriyaki and Kale

Time: 20 minutes

Makes: 2 portions

Prep Time: 10 minutes

Cook Time: 10 minutes

Nutritional Value (per serving):

Net carbs	*6g*
Fat	*53g*
Protein	*38g*
Calories	*675*

Ingredients:

- 2 tbsp gluten-free tamari sauce
- 1 tbsp applesauce
- 2 garlic cloves, minced
- 1 tbsp fresh minced ginger
- 2 beef sirloin steaks, sliced

- 1 tbsp sesame seeds
- 1 tsp sesame oil
- 2 tbsp avocado oil
- 10 white button mushrooms, sliced
- 2 oz curly kale
- Salt and pepper to taste

Directions:

1. Make a marinade by mixing together the ginger, garlic, applesauce, and tamari sauce in a bowl. Place the sliced sirloin steak in the marinade and place it aside.
2. In a pan, fry the sesame seeds until they turn a beautiful golden color.
3. In a frying pan, fry the mushrooms in avocado oil until cooked. Mix in the beef and marinade combination, frying for 2 to 3 minutes. Toward the end, add the kale and cook until the kale wilts.
4. Introduce the sesame oil and salt and pepper to taste and serve.
5. Sprinkle the toasted sesame seeds over your dish and dig in!

Day 5

Breakfast (Optional): Zucchini Bread

Time: 1 hour and 15 minutes

Makes: 10 Slices

Prep Time: 15 minutes

Cook Time: 50 minutes

Nutritional Value (per slice):

Net carbs	1g
Fat	15g
Protein	4g
Calories	162

Ingredients:

- 4 medium eggs
- 1 large zucchini, shredded (moisture squeezed out)
- ½ cup almond flour
- ¼ cup coconut flour
- 8 tbsp coconut oil
- 1 tsp baking powder
- 1 tsp vanilla extract
- Pinch of salt

Directions:

1. While the oven is preheating to 350°F, combine all the ingredients in a bowl.
2. Pour the well-combined ingredients into a bread pan, place it in the oven, and cook for 50 minutes.
3. Allow your bread to cool down before serving. Store the remainder of your bread for a delicious keto-friendly French toast breakfast!

Lunch: Pan-Fried Turkey, Bacon, and Vegetables

Time: 25 minutes

Makes: 2 servings

Prep Time: 10 minutes

Cook Time: 15 minutes

Nutritional Value (per serving):

Net carbs	*3g*
Fat	*52g*
Protein	*47g*
Calories	*665*

Ingredients:

- 3 tbsp coconut oil to cook with
- ¾ lb turkey breast, diced or ground
- 4 slices bacon, diced
- ½ medium onion
- 3 spears asparagus, chopped
- 1 cup spinach, chopped
- 4 tsp fresh thyme, chopped
- Salt and pepper to taste

Directions:

1. Using a pan or a skillet over medium-high heat, melt the coconut oil and fry the diced turkey and bacon for 5 to 7 minutes or until it turns golden in color.

2. Combine the fresh thyme, spinach, asparagus, and onions with the meat and cook everything for an additional 10 minutes to allow the turkey to cook through and the vegetables to soften up.
3. Dust with salt and pepper to taste before serving.

Dinner: Spicy Keto Chili

Time: 1 hour and 15 minutes

Makes: 4 servings

Prep Time: 15 minutes

Cook Time: 1 hour

Nutritional Value (per serving):

Net carbs	*8g*
Fat	*35g*
Protein	*21g*
Calories	*454*

Ingredients:

- 3 tbsp avocado oil to cook with
- 1 medium onion, chopped
- 2 medium bell peppers, diced
- 10 white button mushrooms, chopped
- 1 lb ground beef
- 1 tsp cayenne pepper
- 2 tsp cumin powder

- 1 tsp ground coriander
- 2 tomatoes, diced
- 2 cups beef broth
- 3 cloves garlic, peeled and chopped
- Salt and pepper to taste
- Chopped parsley for garnish

Directions:

1. Sauté bell peppers, chopped onions, and mushrooms in a big pot before introducing the ground beef and all the spices. Cook until the beef has turned brown.
2. Pour the tomato and beef stock into the delicious vegetable and meat mixture and bring it to boil before turning the heat down to medium-low. Partially cover the pot with a lid and allow it to slowly boil for 45 to 50 minutes.
3. If you notice that the mixture is too runny, turn the heat up to medium and allow it to cook uncovered for a few more minutes.
4. Season with chopped garlic and salt and pepper to taste. Garnish with parsley, and enjoy!

Day 6

Breakfast (Optional): Chocolate Hazelnut Muffins

Time: 30 minutes

Makes: 12 muffins

Prep Time: 10 minutes

Cook Time: 20 minutes

Nutritional Value (per muffin):

Net carbs	*3g*
Fat	*25g*
Protein	*8g*
Calories	*282*

Ingredients:
- 3 cups almond flour
- ½ cup melted coconut oil
- 4 large eggs, whisked
- ½ tsp nutmeg
- ¼ tsp cloves
- ½ cup hazelnuts, chopped
- Low-carb sweetener (stevia)
- Pinch of salt
- 1 tsp baking soda
- 3 oz 100% dark chocolate, broken into chunks

Directions:

1. While the oven is preheating to 350°F, combine the baking soda, salt, sweetener, chopped hazelnuts, cloves, nutmeg, eggs, coconut oil, and almond flour.
2. Pour the combination into 12 greased muffin pans and insert the chocolate chunks into the dough.
3. Pop them into the oven for 20 minutes or until a toothpick comes out clean.
4. Allow your muffins to cool down before serving and storing to enjoy again at a later time!

Lunch: Lemony Pepper Tuna Salad

Time: 10 minutes

Makes: 1 serving

Prep Time: 10 minutes

Nutritional Value (per serving):

Net carbs	*11g*
Fat	*40g*
Protein	*45g*
Calories	*480*

Ingredients:

- ⅓ cucumber, diced
- ½ avocado, diced
- 1 tsp lemon juice

- 1 can tuna
- 1 tbsp paleo mayonnaise
- 1 tbsp mustard
- Salt and pepper to taste
- Salad greens

Directions:
1. Combine the avocado, cucumber, and lemon juice.
2. Stir the mayonnaise and mustard into the flaked tuna and add salt and pepper to taste.
3. Mix the tuna and lemony avocado and cucumber.
4. Lay the salad greens in a bowl and scoop the delicious tuna, avocado, and cucumber mixture on top to serve. You can drizzle your salad with olive oil if desired.

Dinner: Apple Dijon Pork Chops (serve with broccoli if desired)

Time: 15 minutes

Makes: 2 servings

Prep Time: 5 minutes

Cook Time: 10 minutes

Nutritional Value (per serving):

Net carbs	4g
Fat	35g
Protein	34g
Calories	450

Ingredients:

- 2 pork chops
- 4 tbsp coconut oil
- 4 tbsp applesauce
- 2 tbsp Dijon mustard
- Salt and pepper to taste

Directions:

1. Mix the applesauce and Dijon mustard in a bowl and place it aside.
2. Rub the pork chops with salt and pepper before heating the coconut oil in a pan on high heat. Place the pork chops in the pan, and cook each side for 3 to 4 minutes or until it has browned.
3. Pour the applesauce and Dijon mustard mixture over the chops and serve. You can opt for roasted broccoli or salad greens on the side.

Day 7

Breakfast (Optional): Frothy Bulletproof Coffee

Time: 2 minutes

Makes: 1 cup

Prep Time: 2 minutes

Nutritional Value (per serving):

Net carbs	*0g*
Fat	*22g*
Protein	*0g*
Calories	*190*

Ingredients:

- 1 cup black coffee
- ½ tbsp coconut oil
- 1 tbsp ghee
- 2 tbsp unsweetened coconut or almond milk

Directions:

1. Blend or use a milk frother to mix all the ingredients.
2. Mix until you see froth forming, serve, and enjoy.

Lunch: Caesar Salad With Garlic Shrimp

Time: 25 minutes

Makes: 4 servings

Prep Time: 15 minutes

Cook Time: 10 minutes

Nutritional Value (per serving):

Net carbs	*5g*
Fat	*19g*
Protein	*25g*
Calories	*296*

Ingredients for the shrimp:
- 1 lb shrimp (shell removed)
- 2 tbsp olive oil
- 1 tbsp lemon juice
- 3 tbsp garlic powder
- 1 tbsp onion powder
- Salt and pepper to taste

Ingredients for the salad:
- 1 head romaine lettuce, chopped
- 1 cucumber, chopped into cubes

Ingredients for the dressing:

- 1 tsp Dijon mustard
- ¼ cup paleo mayonnaise
- 1 tbsp fresh lemon juice
- 2 tsp garlic powder
- Salt and pepper to taste

Garnish:

- 1 tbsp chopped parsley
- 1 tbsp sliced almonds

Directions:

1. While the oven is preheating to 400°F, combine the onion powder, garlic, lemon juice, olive oil, and shrimp together. Season with salt and pepper to taste. Place the combination on a baking tray and cook it in the oven for 10 minutes.
2. While your shrimp is cooking, mix the garlic powder, lemon juice, mustard, mayonnaise, salt, and pepper to make the dressing.
3. Remove the shrimp from the oven and allow them to cool for a few minutes before tossing all the elements together.
4. Garnish your spectacular salad with parsley and chopped almonds, and serve.

Dinner: Pan-Fried Pork Tenderloin With Garlic Spinach

Time: 25 minutes

Makes: 2 servings

Prep Time: 5 minutes

Cook Time: 20 minutes

Nutritional Value (per serving):

Net carbs	0g
Fat	15g
Protein	47g
Calories	330

Ingredients:

- 1 lb pork tenderloin
- Salt and pepper to taste
- 2 tbsp coconut oil to cook with
- 1 ½ cup chopped spinach
- 1 clove garlic, minced

Directions:

1. Slice the tenderloin into two equal halves.
2. Pour the coconut oil into a pan to melt on medium heat and add the tenderloin to the pan to allow it to fry. Using tongs, keep turning the pork to cook evenly on all sides.
3. Cook it until it shows an internal temperature of just below 145°F (it will still cook a little after you've removed it from the pan).
4. Allow the pork to rest for a few minutes before slicing it into 1-inch-thick slices.
5. In the same pan, fry the spinach and garlic for a few minutes or until the spinach has wilted slightly and serve it as a side dish.

Day 8

Breakfast (Optional): Breakfast Stack

Time: 30 minutes

Makes: 2 servings

Prep Time: 15 minutes

Cook Time: 15 minutes

Nutritional Value (per serving):

Net carbs	*5g*
Fat	*54g*
Protein	*38g*
Calories	*680*

Ingredients:
- 4 slices bacon
- ¼ lb ground pork
- ¼ lb ground chicken
- 2 tsp Italian seasoning
- 1 egg, whisked
- 1 tsp salt
- ¼ tsp black pepper
- 2 large portobello mushrooms
- 1 avocado, sliced

Directions:
1. Crisp the bacon and leave the rendered fat in the pan.
2. In a bowl, blend the salt, egg, and Italian seasoning with the chicken and ground pork and make 4 thin patties.
3. Place the patties in the pan with bacon fat and fry until cooked. Remove them from the pan and place them aside.
4. Put the portobello mushrooms in the pan and cook them for 2 to 3 minutes.
5. Place the mushrooms at the bottom on a plate and top each with 2 patties, 3 slices of avocado, and top it off with a slice of bacon.

Lunch: Chicken Cauliflower Couscous Salad

Time: 20 minutes

Makes: 4 servings

Prep Time: 10 minutes

Cook Time: 10 minutes

Nutritional Value (per serving):

Net carbs	*7g*
Fat	*17g*
Protein	*26g*
Calories	*286*

Ingredients:

- 1 lb chicken breast, diced and pan-fried
- 1 tbsp olive oil
- 1 small cauliflower head, grated
- 1 cucumber, diced small
- 1 red pepper, diced small
- 1 tbsp lemon juice
- 2 tbsp olive oil
- 1 cup fresh parsley, finely chopped
- 4 green onions
- 2 tsp garlic powder
- 2 tsp cumin powder
- Salt and pepper to taste

Directions:

1. It's as easy as mixing all these ingredients together and serving!

Dinner: Super Easy Salmon Curry

Time: 25 minutes

Makes: 2 servings

Prep Time: 10 minutes

Cook Time: 15 minutes

Nutritional Value (per serving):

Net carbs	*10g*
Fat	*44g*
Protein	*49g*
Calories	*240*

Ingredients:

- ½ medium onion, diced
- 2 cups green beans, diced
- 1 ½ tbsp curry powder
- 1 tsp garlic powder
- Cream from the top of 1 can of coconut milk
- 2 cups bone broth
- 1 lb raw salmon, diced
- 2 tbsp coconut oil to cook with
- Salt and pepper to taste
- 2 tbsp basil, chopped (for garnish)

Directions:

1. Fry the diced onion in coconut oil until cooked before placing green beans in the pan as well.
2. Pour the broth into the pot and bring it to a boil. Combine the salmon, garlic powder, and curry powder with the broth mixture.
3. Pour the coconut cream into the combination and let it boil on medium-low heat for 3 to 5 minutes. Sprinkle with salt and pepper to taste and garnish your dish with basil.

Day 9

Breakfast (Optional): Blueberry Muffins

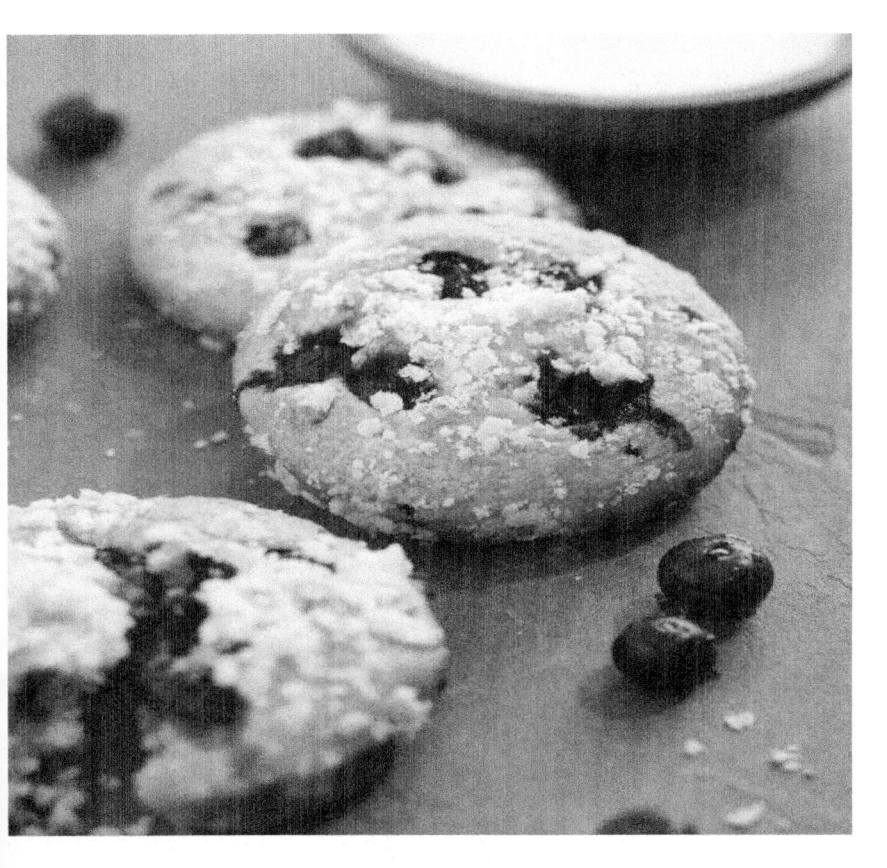

Time: 30 minutes

Makes: 6 servings

Prep Time: 10 minutes

Cook Time: 20 minutes

Nutritional Value (per serving):

Net carbs	3g
Fat	22g
Protein	7g
Calories	240

Ingredients:

- 1 ½ cups almond flour
- ¼ cup ghee, melted
- 2 eggs, whisked
- ½ cup blueberries
- 1 tbsp vanilla extract
- Stevia to taste
- ½ tsp baking soda
- Pinch of salt

Directions:

1. Mix together the eggs, vanilla extract, stevia, salt, baking soda, almond flour, and ghee while you're waiting for the oven to preheat to 350°F.
2. Squeeze the blueberries (so that the skins burst) into the mix and stir well. Save 12 blueberries to top your muffins with.
3. Grease the muffin pan with ghee and scoop the combination into the pan (about ¾ full). Place 2 blueberries on each muffin.
4. Place them in the oven for 20 minutes or until a toothpick comes out clean.
5. Allow your muffins to cool before serving with whipped cream if desired.

Lunch: Mini Ham and Spinach Quiches

Time: 25 minutes

Makes: 4 mini quiches

Serving Size: 2

Prep Time: 10 minutes

Cook Time: 15 minutes

Nutritional Value (per serving):

Net carbs	*3g*
Fat	*13g*
Protein	*20g*
Calories	*210*

Ingredients:

- 3 eggs, whisked
- 4 slices ham, diced
- ¾ cup spinach, chopped
- ¼ cup leek, chopped
- ¼ cup coconut milk
- ½ tsp baking powder
- Salt and pepper to taste

Directions:

1. While the oven is preheating to 450°F, blend all the ingredients together.

2. Pour the combination into 4 tart pans and cook in the oven for 15 minutes or until a toothpick comes out clean.
3. Enjoy this as a delicious lunch or a quick snack.

Dinner: Beef Fajitas

Time: 20 minutes

Makes: 2 servings

Prep Time: 5 minutes

Cook Time: 15 minutes

Nutritional Value (per serving):

Net carbs	*4g*
Fat	*47g*
Protein	*46g*
Calories	*640*

Ingredients:
- ½ medium onion, chopped
- 1 bell pepper, chopped
- 1 lb beef, sliced into strips (choose a steak of your choice)
- 2 tbsp coconut oil to cook with
- 1 tbsp cumin powder
- 1 tbsp garlic powder
- 1 tbsp onion powder
- A pinch of chili powder
- 1 tbsp cilantro, finely chopped

- Salt and pepper to taste
- Romaine lettuce leaves (optional)

Directions:

1. Melt the coconut oil in a pan and fry the chopped onions and bell pepper until cooked.
2. In a separate pan, fry the steak strips. Once the onions have turned translucent, add the beef strips to the onion and bell pepper combination and season it with cumin powder, garlic powder, onion powder, a pinch of chili powder, and chopped cilantro. Add salt and pepper to taste. Cook it for 2 more minutes and serve immediately. Make a scrumptious wrap by filling lettuce leaves with the meat mixture.

Day 10

Breakfast (Optional): Collagen Booster Coffee

Time: 5 minutes

Makes: 1 cup

Prep Time: 5 minutes

Nutritional Value (per serving):

Net carbs	0g
Fat	14g
Protein	5g
Calories	160

Ingredients:

- 1 cup black coffee
- 1 tbsp ghee
- ½ scoop unflavored hydrolyzed collagen powder

Directions:

1. Using a blender or a milk frother, combine all the ingredients well until you see foam forming.

Lunch: Mini Spinach Meatloaves

Time: 25 minutes

Makes: 12 servings

Prep Time: 5 minutes

Cook Time: 20 minutes

Nutritional Value (per serving):

Net carbs	*5g*
Fat	*30g*
Protein	*30g*
Calories	*430*

Ingredients:

- ¼ lb ground turkey
- ¼ lb ground beef
- ½ small onion, diced
- 2 garlic cloves, minced
- ⅓ lb fresh spinach, chopped finely
- 4 eggs, whisked
- 2 tbsp Italian seasoning
- ½ tbsp salt
- ½ tbsp black pepper
- ⅓ cup almond or coconut milk
- Coconut oil to cook with

Directions:

1. While the oven is preheating to 400°F, fry the diced onions, ground turkey, and garlic in 1 tbsp of coconut oil in a pan. Once the meat is cooked, introduce the spinach and fry it for an additional 1 to 2 minutes. Then, grease the muffin pans with ghee and place them aside.
2. Mix the fried meat mixture with the whisked eggs and season it with Italian seasoning, salt, and pepper. Add the almond or coconut milk to the combination and stir well.

3. Pour the combination into the 12 muffin cups, dividing it equally. Pop them in the oven for 10 minutes or until they've turned solid.

Dinner: Creamy Tomato and Chicken Keto Pasta

Time: 25 minutes

Makes: 2 servings

Prep Time: 10 minutes

Cook Time: 15 minutes

Nutritional Value (per serving):

Net carbs	*9g*
Fat	*27g*
Protein	*59g*
Calories	*540*

Ingredients:
- 2 chicken breasts, cubed
- 2 tbsp ghee or coconut oil to cook with
- 2 tomatoes, diced
- ½ cup basil, finely chopped
- ¼ cup coconut milk
- 6 cloves garlic, minced
- Salt to taste
- 1 zucchini, shredded to resemble noodles

Directions:

1. Sauté the chicken in the ghee until cooked before adding the tomatoes and salt to taste. Reduce the heat to medium-low, and boil the liquid down.
2. Stir the coconut milk, garlic, and basil into the chicken and allow it to slowly boil for a few minutes longer.
3. Divide the pasta between 2 bowls and top it with the delicious creamy chicken mixture.

Day 11

Breakfast (Optional): Apple Cinnamon Muffins

Time: 30 minutes

Makes: 12 muffins

Prep Time: 10 minutes

Cook Time: 20 minutes

Nutritional Value (per muffin):

Net carbs	*3g*
Fat	*22g*
Protein	*7g*
Calories	*241*

Ingredients:

- 3 cups almond flour
- ½ cup ghee, melted
- 3 large eggs, whisked
- 3 tbsp cinnamon
- 1 tsp nutmeg
- ¼ tsp cloves
- 4 tbsp applesauce
- 1 tsp lemon juice
- Stevia to taste
- 1 tsp baking soda

Directions:

1. While the oven is preheating to 350°F, stir all the ingredients together well.
2. Grease silicone muffin pans with ghee before pouring the combination into the muffin pans.
3. Cook them in the oven for approximately 20 minutes or until a toothpick comes out clean.

Lunch: Bacon and Avo Caesar Salad

Time: 15 minutes

Makes: 2 servings

Prep Time: 10 minutes

Cook Time: 5 minutes

Nutritional Value (per serving):

Net carbs	6g
Fat	65g
Protein	10g
Calories	652

Ingredients for the salad:

- 4 slices bacon, diced
- 1 head romaine lettuce, chopped
- ½ cucumber, sliced finely
- ¼ medium onion, diced
- 1 large avocado, sliced

Ingredients for the salad dressing:

- ¼ cup mayonnaise
- 1 tbsp lemon juice
- 1 tsp Dijon mustard
- 1 tsp garlic powder
- Salt and pepper to taste

Directions:

1. Pan-fry the bacon in a nonstick pan until crispy or for approximately 5 minutes. Remove the crispy bacon from the pan and place it aside on a paper towel.
2. Stir the garlic powder, mustard, lemon juice, and mayonnaise together in a bowl and sprinkle it with salt and pepper to taste before combining it with the onions, cucumber, and romaine lettuce leaves.

3. Divide your mixture between 2 bowls and top each with equal amounts of mouthwatering crispy bacon and avocado slices.

Dinner: Pork and Cabbage Stew

Time: 2 hours and 10 minutes

Makes: 4 servings

Prep Time: 10 minutes

Cook Time: 2 hours

Nutritional Value (per serving):

Net carbs	*9g*
Fat	*28g*
Protein	*23g*
Calories	*400*

Ingredients:
- 1 lb pork shoulder (boneless)
- 3 cups cold water
- 1 head cabbage, chopped
- 1 onion or leek, chopped
- 1 large chunk fresh ginger, chopped into large pieces
- 1 tbsp apple cider vinegar
- Salt to taste
- Coconut oil to cook the pork with

Directions:

1. Melt 2 tbsp of coconut oil in a large pot before adding the cubed pork. Fry until the pork is cooked.
2. Stir in the chopped leek, ginger, apple cider vinegar, and chopped cabbage. Sprinkle with 2 tsp of salt and add the water to the pot.
3. Cook the pork mixture with a lid over medium-high heat for 2 hours. Be sure to check that the water does not dry up. You can add more water as needed.
4. Sprinkle with salt to taste and remove the ginger pieces before serving.

Day 12

Breakfast (Optional): Yummy French Pancakes

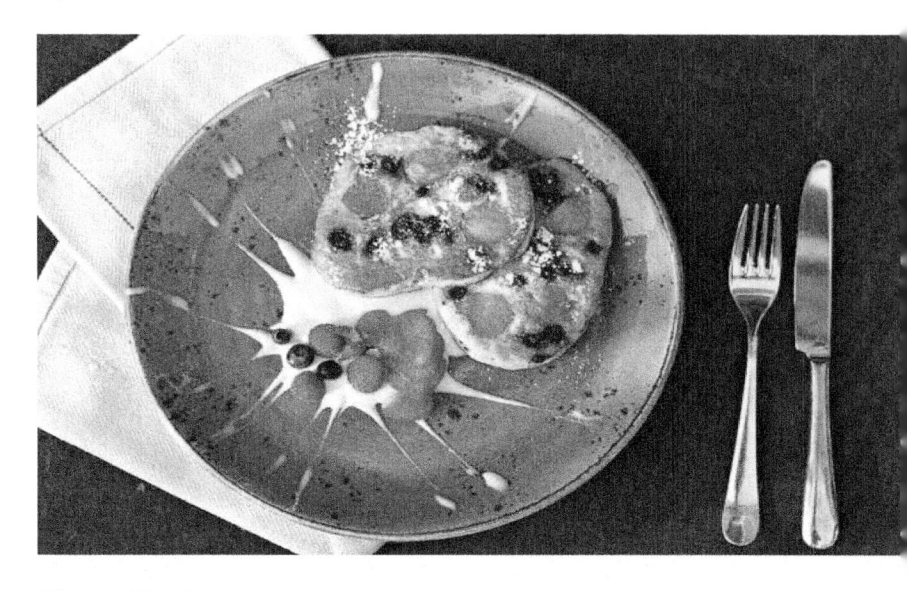

Time: 15 minutes

Makes: 4 servings or 12 pancakes

Serving Size: 3 pancakes

Prep Time: 5 minutes

Cook Time: 10 minutes

Nutritional Value (per serving):

Net carbs	*4g*
Fat	*68g*
Protein	*15g*
Calories	*688*

Ingredients:

- 8 eggs, whisked
- 2 cups heavy whipped cream
- ½ cup water
- ¼ tsp salt
- 2 tbsp ground psyllium powder
- 3 oz ghee
- 4 strawberries, sliced thinly

Directions:

1. Combine the water, cream, eggs, and salt together in a mixing bowl. You can use a hand mixer to combine them well. While doing this, gradually introduce the psyllium husk to the combination until the batter becomes velvety smooth, and then allow it to rest for 10 minutes.
2. After 10 minutes, scoop ½ cup (to make one pancake) of the combination onto a frying pan to cook the pancakes in ghee (just like regular pancakes) on medium heat. Wait until the pancake is dry on top before turning it over to cook on the other side.
3. Serve your pancakes with whipped cream and a few sliced strawberries.

Lunch: Smoked Salmon Ham Wraps With Cucumber

Time: 5 minutes

Makes: 4 servings

Serving Size: 2 wraps

Prep Time: 5 minutes

Nutritional Value (per serving):

Net carbs	*0g*
Fat	*10g*
Protein	*29g*
Calories	*210*

Ingredients:
- 4 slices ham (cooked ham)
- ½ cucumber, cut into thin slices
- 3 ½ oz smoked salmon, sliced
- 1 tbsp coconut cream
- Green salad to serve with

Directions:
1. Lay out the slices of ham and spread them with coconut cream.
2. Put the salmon slices on top of the spread coconut cream.
3. Then, add the cucumber slices on top of the salmon.
4. Roll the ham parcels up and serve them with a side of green salad.

Dinner: Roast Beef With Carrots and Onions

Time: 1 hour and 10 minutes

Makes: 4 servings

Prep Time: 10 minutes

Cook Time: 1 hour

Nutritional Value (per serving):

Net carbs	*5g*
Fat	*62g*
Protein	*38g*
Calories	*379*

Ingredients:

- 2 lbs beef round
- 2 carrots, peeled and roughly chopped
- 1 medium onion, peeled and roughly chopped
- 6 cloves garlic, minced
- 4 tbsp olive oil
- 1 large sprig rosemary
- 1 sprig thyme
- Salt and pepper to taste

Directions:

1. While you're waiting for the oven to preheat to 400°F, combine the garlic, onions, carrots, and olive oil in a baking tray. Place

some of the rosemary and thyme in the mixture and sprinkle with salt.
2. Rub the beef with the remainder of the rosemary, thyme, and salt and put it on top of the vegetables.
3. Pop the tray in the oven and allow it to cook for 1 hour.

Day 13

Breakfast: Eggs Benedict With Mug Bread

Time: 30 minutes

Makes: 2 servings

Prep Time: 15 minutes

Cook Time: 15 minutes

Nutritional Value (per serving):

Net carbs	*3g*
Fat	*58g*
Protein	*15g*
Calories	*590*

Ingredients for the mug bread:
- 1 tsp ghee
- 1 tbsp almond flour
- 1 tbsp coconut flour

- ¾ tsp baking powder
- Pinch of salt
- 1 egg
- 1 tbsp heavy whipped cream

Ingredients for the hollandaise sauce:

- 3 oz ghee
- 2 egg yolks
- 1 tbsp water
- 1 tbsp lemon juice
- Salt and pepper
- A pinch of cayenne pepper (optional, though highly recommended)

Ingredients for the poached eggs:

- 1 tbsp white vinegar (5%)
- Water
- 2 eggs

For serving:

- 1 tbsp butter for frying
- 1 oz smoked deli ham
- 1 tbsp microgreens

Directions for the mug bread:

1. Grease a flat-bottomed mug with ghee before combining all the dry ingredients in the mug with a fork or a spoon.
2. Add the eggs and combine the mixture well before folding in the cream until the mixture is velvety and lump-free.
3. Pop it in the microwave on high for approximately 2 minutes or until a toothpick comes out clean.

4. Allow your mug bread to cool before removing it from the cup and slicing it in half.

Directions for the hollandaise sauce:

1. Melt the butter in a microwave using a cup, and let it cool for a few minutes.
2. Combine the egg yolks and water in a small pot and create a double boiler with a slightly bigger pot underneath. On medium-low heat, stir the mixture regularly until it starts to thicken.
3. Lightly beat the butter into the egg yolks and water mixture, stirring constantly. Add your cayenne pepper, pepper, salt, and lemon, and set it aside.

Directions for the poached eggs:

1. Pour water and vinegar into a saucepan and bring it to a simmer. Make sure the water does not start boiling.
2. One by one, crack your eggs into a cup and slowly pour them into the water. Let each cook for 3 minutes.
3. Remove the eggs carefully with a spoon and place them into cold water before putting the eggs on a plate (you're welcome to trim the rough edges).

Serving:

1. Place your mug bread halves in a frying pan with butter on medium-high heat for a few minutes.
2. Remove them from the pan and place them on a plate. Top each half with smoked ham, then the poached egg, and drizzle with hollandaise sauce.
3. Garnish your eggs benedict with watercress if desired, and enjoy!

Lunch: Blueberry Chaffels

Time: 21 minutes

Makes: 4 servings

Serving Size: 4 chaffels

Prep Time: 15 minutes

Cook Time: 6 minutes

Nutritional Value (per serving):

Net carbs	*10g*
Fat	*22g*
Protein	*13g*
Calories	*293*

Ingredients for the blueberry chaffels:
- 4 eggs
- 1 cup shredded mozzarella cheese
- 1 tbsp coconut flour
- 1 tsp vanilla extract
- 3 oz fresh blueberries

Serving:
- ½ cup heavy whipping cream
- 6 oz blueberries

Directions:

1. While the waffle maker is preheating, combine the eggs, mozzarella cheese, coconut flour, vanilla extract, and fresh blueberries in a mixing bowl. Stir the ingredients well and set the bowl aside for 5 minutes to allow the coconut flour to absorb moisture.
2. In your greased waffle maker, evenly spread the batter on the bottom plate with a spoon, close it, and allow it to cook for 6 minutes (depending on your waffle maker).
3. Serve your waffle with heavy whipping cream and fresh blueberries.

Dinner: Cheesy Meatballs (Italian Style)

Time: 50 minutes

Makes: 4 servings

Prep Time: 20 minutes

Cook Time: 30 minutes

Nutritional Value (per serving):

Net carbs	*5g*
Fat	*49g*
Protein	*39g*
Calories	*628*

Ingredients:

- 1 lb ground beef or ground turkey
- ¾ cup shredded Parmesan cheese
- 1 egg
- 1 tsp salt
- ½ tbsp dried basil
- ½ tsp onion powder
- 1 tsp garlic powder
- ½ tsp ground black pepper
- 3 tbsp olive oil
- 1 lb whole tomato
- 2 tbsp fresh parsley, finely chopped
- 7 oz fresh spinach
- 2 oz ghee
- 5 oz fresh mozzarella cheese
- A pinch of salt and pepper

Directions:

1. Combine the spices, egg, Parmesan cheese, ground beef, and salt in a bowl and stir well.
2. Make balls with the combination (1 oz each, roughly), making sure to keep your hands wet to prevent the meatballs from sticking.
3. Fry the meatballs in a pan with olive oil until they've turned brown on all sides.
4. Turn the heat down and add the fresh tomatoes. Allow the combination to slowly boil for approximately 15 minutes and make sure that you stir it occasionally. Spice it up with salt and pepper to taste and some parsley and stir. If you wish to freeze this delicious dish to enjoy on another day, scoop it into a bowl and allow it to cool down before freezing.

5. In a separate pan, melt ghee and fry the spinach for 1 to 2 minutes and add salt and pepper as desired. Add the spinach to the meatball mixture and mix well.
6. Serve your dish topped with either shredded or torn mozzarella.

Day 14

Breakfast: Classic Bacon and Eggs

Time: 10 minutes

Makes: 4 servings

Prep Time: 2 minutes

Cook Time: 8 minutes

Nutritional Value (per serving):

Net carbs	*2g*
Fat	*31g*
Protein	*33g*
Calories	*425*

Ingredients:
- 8 eggs
- 9 oz bacon slices
- Cherry tomatoes (optional)

- Fresh thyme (optional)

Directions:

1. Render the bacon fat by frying it until crispy on medium-high heat. Place the bacon aside and keep the fat in the pan.
2. Break the eggs into the bacon-greased pan and fry them to your liking.
3. Cut the cherry tomatoes in half and fry them with the eggs.
4. Garnish your eggs with fresh chopped thyme and serve.

Lunch: Seafood Chowder

Time: 40 minutes

Makes: 4 servings

Prep Time: 20 minutes

Cook Time: 20 minutes

Nutritional Value (per serving):

Net carbs	*6g*
Fat	*69g*
Protein	*37g*
Calories	*792*

Ingredients:

- 4 tbsp ghee
- 2 cloves garlic, minced
- 5 oz celery stalk, chopped

- 1 cup clam juice
- 1 ½ cup heavy whipping cream
- 2 tsp dried sage or dried thyme
- ½ lemon, juiced and zest
- 4 oz cream cheese
- 1 lb salmon fillets (or any other firm fish), cubed
- 2 oz baby spinach
- 8 oz shrimp, peeled and deveined
- Salt and ground black pepper
- ½ tbsp red chili pepper, chopped
- Fresh sage (optional for garnish)

Directions:

1. Using a large pot, melt the butter on medium heat and then add the garlic and celery. Fry for 5 minutes, then add the lemon zest, lemon juice, sage, cream cheese, cream, and clam juice to the pot and allow it to boil for 10 minutes uncovered.
2. Introduce your fish to the combination and allow it to boil for another 3 minutes or until the fish flakes easily. Then, add the baby spinach leaves and let cook until slightly wilted.
3. Spice it up with your desired amount of salt and pepper.
4. You can garnish your dish with red chili pepper and fresh sage for a beautiful splash of color and an intense burst of flavor.

Dinner: Bacon and Mushroom Casserole

Time: 55 minutes

Makes: 4 servings

Prep Time: 10 minutes

Cook Time: 45 minutes

Nutritional Value (per serving):

Net carbs	6g
Fat	78g
Protein	46g
Calories	914

Ingredients:

- 6 oz mushroom, cut into quarters
- 6 oz diced bacon
- 2 oz ghee
- 8 eggs
- 1 cup heavy whipping cream
- 1 ¼ cup shredded cheddar cheese
- 1 tsp onion powder
- Salt and pepper to taste

Directions:

1. While the oven is preheating to 400°F, start frying the bacon and mushrooms in a nonstick pan on medium-high heat until it develops a honey-brown color. Add salt and pepper as desired.
2. Grease a baking dish, and add the fried elements to the dish.
3. In a bowl, combine the eggs, whipping cream, shredded cheddar cheese, and onion powder together and season it with salt and pepper.
4. Pour the combination over the bacon and mushrooms, and cook it in the oven for 30 to 40 minutes or until set.
5. You can cover the dish with aluminum foil to prevent the top from burning before the dish is cooked through.

Chapter 5:

A 12-Day Meal Plan With Recipes for Vegetarians

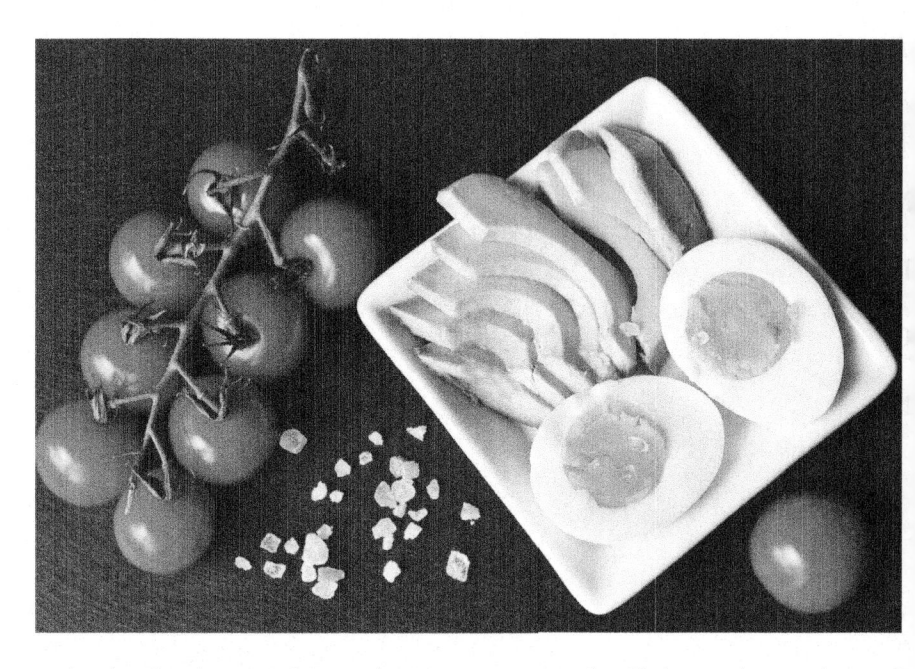

It is absolutely possible to be vegetarian and still have the option of delicious keto-friendly meals. These recipes include great substitutions for meat, such as eggs and cheese, and will keep you feeling satisfied and full! You'll get to pick and choose on which days you want to eat certain meals, so the following meal plans are just an example of what your diet should look like.

Feel free to mix and match breakfasts, lunches, and dinners according to the time you have available to cook. These meals are highly nutritious and wholesome, and they're sure to tickle your tastebuds and curb cravings. Take some time over a weekend or on days that aren't too crazy to prepare your meals in advance. You can store or freeze some of these meals to avoid cooking all week, to grab an easy breakfast, or to pack a healthy lunchbox to enjoy at work.

Day 1

Breakfast (Optional): Strawberry Smoothie

Time: 5 minutes

Makes: 2 servings

Prep Time: 3 minutes

Cook Time: 2 minutes

Nutritional Value (per serving):

Net carbs	*10g*
Fat	*42g*
Protein	*4g*
Calories	*416*

Ingredients:

- 1 ¾ cup unsweetened coconut milk
- 5 oz fresh strawberries, sliced
- 1 tbsp lime juice
- ½ tsp vanilla extract

Directions:
1. Using a blender, combine all the ingredients. For a deliciously creamy smoothie, drain all the liquid from the can of coconut milk before use. You can add more lime juice if desired. If you crave a dairy smoothie, feel free to substitute the coconut milk with 1 ¼ cup of Greek yogurt.

Lunch: Delicious Deviled Eggs

Time: 20 minutes

Makes: 6 servings

Serving Size: 2 pieces

Prep Time: 10 minutes

Cook Time: 10 minutes

Nutritional Value (per serving):

Net carbs	*1g*
Fat	*18g*
Protein	*6g*
Calories	*197*

Ingredients:
- 6 eggs
- 1 tbsp red curry paste (you may use chipotle paste or any other chili paste)
- ½ cup mayonnaise (you may use vegan mayonnaise)

- ¼ tsp salt
- ½ tbsp poppy seeds

Directions:

1. Using a pot, place the eggs in cold water. Use just enough water to cover the eggs and bring them to a boil uncovered. Allow them to boil for 8 minutes and then quickly place them in an ice bath.
2. Remove them from the ice bath, de-shell your eggs, and cut them in half. Using a spoon, remove the egg yolks and put them in a bowl, and place the egg whites on a plate in the fridge.
3. Combine the curry paste, mayonnaise, and egg yolks until it forms a velvety batter, then add salt to taste.
4. Remove the egg whites from the fridge. Scoop the egg yolk batter into the hollowed egg whites, and sprinkle them with poppy seeds before serving.

Dinner: Goat Cheese and Spinach Pie

Time: 70 minutes

Makes: 6 servings

Prep Time: 30 minutes

Cook Time: 40 minutes

Nutritional Value (per serving):

Net carbs	4g
Fat	57g
Protein	23g
Calories	636

Ingredients for the pie crust:

- 1 ¼ cup almond flour
- 3 tbsp sesame seeds
- 1 tbsp ground psyllium husk
- ½ tsp salt
- 1 ½ oz butter
- 1 egg

Ingredients for the egg batter:

- 5 eggs
- 1 cup heavy whipping cream or sour cream
- Salt and pepper to taste

Ingredients for the filling:

- 6 ½ cups spinach, chopped
- 2 tbsp butter or coconut oil
- 1 clove garlic, finely chopped
- 1 pinch ground nutmeg
- Salt and pepper
- 1 cup cheddar cheese, shredded
- 1 ½ cup goat cheese, sliced

Directions:

1. While you're waiting for the oven to preheat to 350°F, combine the almond flour and sesame seeds using a blender. Introduce the psyllium husk, butter, egg, and salt to form a dough. Press the dough into a cake pan, and use a fork to make holes in the dough on the bottom of the pan.
2. Pop the pie shell in the oven for 10 to 15 minutes, and start to stir together the eggs and whipping cream (or sour cream). Sprinkle with salt and pepper as desired and set it aside.
3. Use a pan to fry the garlic in butter (or coconut oil), then add the spinach to the pan and fry it for 2 minutes or until the spinach has wilted slightly. Sprinkle with salt and pepper as desired.
4. Remove the pie shell from the oven and pour the spinach mixture into the shell. Stir the cheddar cheese into your egg mixture and pour it over the spinach. Top the mixture with goat cheese slices.
5. Pop your pan back into the oven for another 30 to 40 minutes.

Day 2

Breakfast (Optional): Buttery Basil Scrambled Eggs

Time: 10 minutes

Makes: 1 serving

Prep Time: 5 minutes

Cook Time: 5 minutes

Nutritional Value (per serving):

Net carbs	3g
Fat	61g
Protein	25g
Calories	657

Ingredients:

- 2 tbsp butter
- 2 eggs
- 2 tbsp heavy whipping cream
- Salt and pepper
- ½ cup cheddar cheese, grated
- 2 tbsp fresh basil

Directions:

1. Use a pan on low heat to melt the butter. While you're waiting for the butter to melt, crack the eggs into a bowl and stir in the cheddar cheese, cream, and salt and pepper as desired.
2. Pour your egg mixture into the pan and fold it continuously with a spatula until cooked or to your liking.
3. Top your eggs with fresh basil before serving.

Lunch: Cauliflower Hash Browns

Time: 40 minutes

Makes: 4 servings

Prep Time: 10 minutes

Cook Time: 30 minutes

Nutritional Value (per serving):

Net carbs	*5g*
Fat	*26g*
Protein	*7g*
Calories	*282*

Ingredients:

- 1 lb cauliflower
- 3 eggs
- ½ yellow onion, grated
- 1 tsp salt
- 2 pinches pepper
- 4 oz butter to cook with

Directions:

1. Rinse and trim the cauliflower. Then, use a grater to grate the cauliflower. Put the grated cauliflower in a bowl and combine it with the eggs, onion, and salt and pepper as desired. Set the combination aside for 5 to 10 minutes.

2. Melt the butter in a nonstick pan over medium heat. Use a spoon to place the cauliflower in the pan and press down on it to form a patty. You can do three or four at a time to speed up the cooking process.
3. Cook each patty for 4 to 5 minutes per side. Make sure to adjust the heat as necessary to prevent them from burning. Be patient with the cooking process as flipping them over too quickly can make them fall apart.
4. Serve your delicious cauliflower hash browns with a side of leafy green salad for a burst of color and crunch.

Dinner: Homemade Pesto Gnocchi

Time: 55 minutes

Makes: 4 servings

Prep Time: 40 minutes

Cook Time: 15 minutes

Nutritional Value (per serving):

Net carbs	*6g*
Fat	*80g*
Protein	*32g*
Calories	*881*

Ingredients:

- ½ lb cauliflower
- ¾ cup shredded Parmesan cheese

- 1 cup almond flour
- 2 egg yolks
- 1 tsp onion powder (optional)
- 1 tsp ground psyllium husk powder
- ½ tsp salt
- 1 cup shredded cheese (cheddar or mozzarella)
- 1 tbsp olive oil or ghee

Ingredients for the pesto:

- ½ cup olive oil (divided)
- ¾ cup Parmesan cheese
- 2 oz pine nuts
- 1 oz fresh basil
- 1 clove garlic
- Salt and pepper to taste

Directions:

1. After you've washed and cleaned the cauliflower, break it into small florets. Steam the florets for a few minutes and then blend them using a food processor until it forms a velvety smooth texture. Dry the cauliflower by placing the smooth puree in a paper towel and squeezing out the moisture (the drier, the better).
2. Put the cauliflower back into the food processor with the almond flour, egg yolks, onion powder, psyllium husk powder, and olive oil. Beat the combination until it's combined well.
3. In a pan over medium-low heat, melt the cheese gently (make sure you stir it constantly) and introduce the melted cheese to the mixture in the food processor and beat until the mixture forms a soft dough.
4. Make long rolls per person (4) and put the rolls in the fridge for an hour.

5. Remove the rolls from the fridge and break them into pieces to make small balls (12).
6. In a pan, melt butter on medium-high heat and add the gnocchi. Allow them to cook until warm and light brown.
7. Combine the ingredients for the pesto with half of the olive oil in a food processor for a few minutes. Then, introduce the rest of the oil and beat it for a few more minutes.
8. Toss the gnocchi with your homemade pesto and serve with a dash of Parmesan cheese on top.

Day 3

Breakfast (Optional): Easy Mexican-Style Eggs

Time: 1 hour

Makes: 4 servings

Prep Time: 15 minutes

Cook Time: 45 minutes

Nutritional Value (per serving):

Net carbs	12g
Fat	47g
Protein	17g
Calories	547

Ingredients:

- ½ cup olive oil
- 1 white onion, grated
- 2 cloves garlic, minced
- 2 fresh jalapeños, diced
- 2 cups crushed tomatoes
- 2 tsp salt
- 1 tsp pepper
- 8 eggs

To serve:

- ½ cup shredded queso fresco
- 4 tbsp fresh cilantro, chopped
- 1 avocado, sliced

Directions:

1. Heat ⅓ of the olive oil over medium heat and fry the jalapeños until they turn soft. Once the jalapeños are soft, put the onions and garlic in the pan and fry them until the onions turn translucent.
2. Add in the tomatoes and reduce the heat. Allow them to cook covered until the mixture turns thick. Add salt and pepper to taste, remove the pan from the heat and place it aside.
3. In a frying pan, use the remainder of the oil to fry the eggs to your liking. Season your eggs with salt and pepper as desired.
4. Scoop the tomato mixture into a bowl and place two eggs on top. Garnish your dish with queso fresco and cilantro. Serve your delicious spicy dish with avocado slices on the side and enjoy!

Lunch: A Simple Greek Salad

Time: 10 minutes

Makes: 2 servings

Prep Time: 10 minutes

Nutritional Value (per serving):

Net carbs	*15g*
Fat	*51g*
Protein	*17g*
Calories	*590*

Ingredients:
- 3 ripe tomatoes
- ½ cucumber
- ½ red onion
- ½ green bell pepper
- 7 oz feta cheese
- 10 black Greek olives
- ¼ cup olive oil
- ½ tbsp red wine vinegar
- Salt and pepper to taste
- 2 tsp dried oregano

Directions:
1. Slice the tomatoes, cucumber, onion, and bell pepper into bite-sized pieces. Plate the salad as desired and sprinkle it with feta

cheese and olives. Drizzle the olive oil and vinegar over your salad.
2. Serve with salt and pepper as desired and a dash of dried oregano.

Dinner: Rich and Creamy Broccoli and Leek Soup

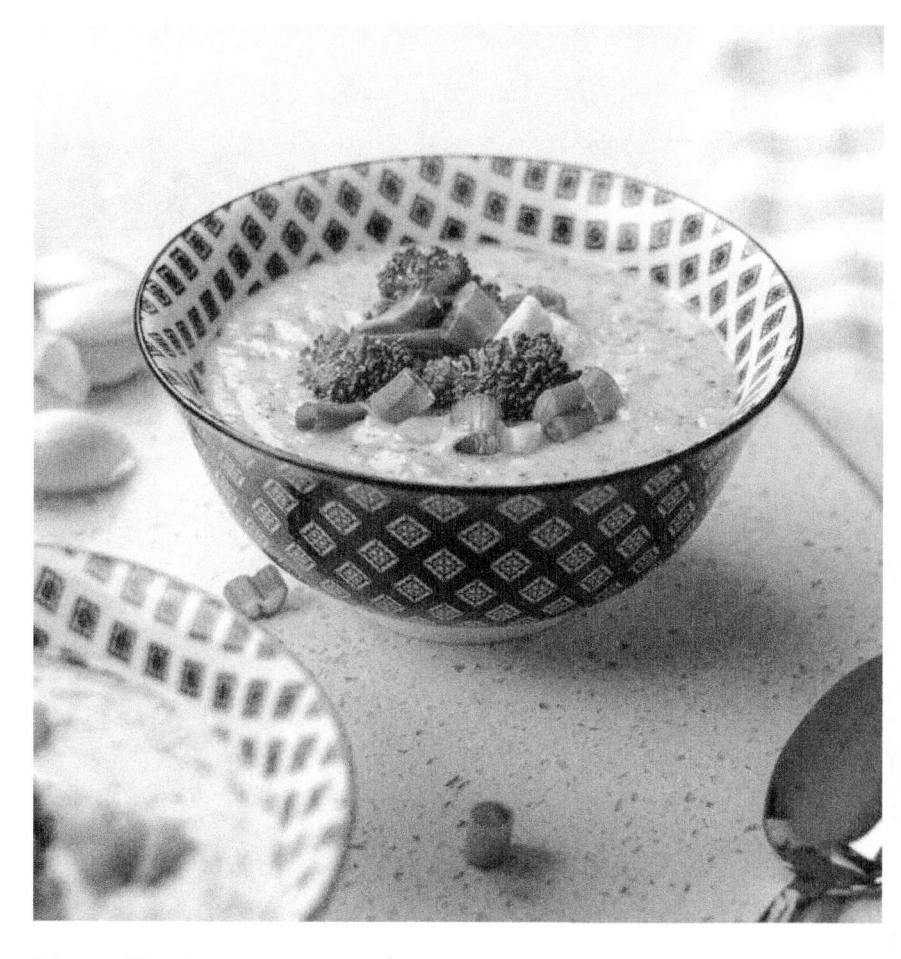

Time: 20 minutes

Makes: 4 servings

Prep Time: 5 minutes

Cook Time: 15 minutes

Nutritional Value (per serving):

Net carbs	11g
Fat	53g
Protein	17g
Calories	588

Ingredients for the soup:

- 1 leek
- ⅔ lb broccoli
- 2 cups water
- 1 vegetable bouillon cube
- 7 oz cream cheese
- 1 cup heavy whipping cream
- ½ tsp ground black pepper
- ½ cup fresh basil, chopped
- 1 clove garlic, minced

Ingredients for the cheese chips:

- 1 ½ cup shredded cheddar cheese
- ½ tsp paprika powder

Directions for the soup:

1. Chop the whole leek after you've rinsed it. Remove the core of the broccoli and slice it thinly. Break the head of broccoli into small florets and set it aside.
2. Using a big pot on high heat, boil the thinly sliced broccoli core and chopped leek with salt and the bouillon cube for a few minutes or until they can be easily pierced with a knife. Then, introduce the broccoli florets and reduce the heat. Allow the mixture to boil until the florets are tender.

3. Stir in the garlic, basil, ground pepper, cream cheese, and cream. Use a stick blender to achieve the desired consistency. If the soup is too thick, you can add some water. If you'd like a thicker consistency, add a dash of cream.

Directions for the cheese chips:
1. While the oven is preheating to 400°F, line a large baking pan with parchment paper. Grate the cheese and use a tablespoon to scoop small heaps onto the parchment paper (space them 1 inch apart).
2. Dust the heaps of cheese with paprika and bake them in the oven for 5 to 6 minutes.
3. You can sprinkle your cheese heaps with different types of herbs or spices for different flavored chips. Enjoy them as a snack or a side to just about any soup.

Day 4

Breakfast (Optional): Blueberry Smoothie

Time: 5 minutes

Makes: 2 servings

Prep Time: 5 minutes

Nutritional Value (per serving):

Net carbs	9g
Fat	32g
Protein	3g
Calories	323

Ingredients:

- 1 ⅓ cup unsweetened coconut milk
- 3 oz fresh blueberries
- 1 tbsp lemon juice
- ½ tsp vanilla extract

Directions:

1. Using a blender, combine all the ingredients together.
2. You can add more lemon juice if desired. Feel free to use Greek yogurt instead of coconut milk for a thicker dairy smoothie.

Lunch: Swedish Turnip Fritters

Time: 30 minutes

Makes: 4 servings

Prep Time: 10 minutes

Cook Time: 20 minutes

Nutritional Value (per serving):

Net carbs	12g
Fat	66g
Protein	23g
Calories	756

Ingredients for the turnips:
- 1 lb Swedish turnips
- 8 oz Halloumi cheese
- 4 eggs
- 3 tbsp coconut flour
- A pinch of turmeric
- 1 tsp salt
- ¼ tsp pepper
- 2 oz ghee to cook with

Ingredients for the ranch mayonnaise:
- ½ cup mayonnaise
- 1 tbsp ranch seasoning

For serving:
- 2 avocados
- 5 oz leafy greens

Directions:
1. While the oven is preheating to 250°F, wash and peel the Swedish turnips. Grate the turnips and the cheese.
2. In a bowl, combine the coconut flour, eggs, turmeric, cheese, Swedish turnips, and salt and pepper to taste. Allow it to rest

for 3 to 5 minutes so that the coconut flour can absorb the moisture.
3. Melt the butter in a frying pan over medium-high heat. Make 3 very thin (⅛ inches) patties per serving with the turnip combination and place them in the pan to cook. If they are too thick, the turnip won't cook through.
4. Fry the turnip patties for approximately 3 to 5 minutes per side. You can place the patties in the oven to keep them warm for serving.
5. Combine the ranch seasoning with mayonnaise.
6. Serve your delicious fritters with a dash of ranch mayo and a side of leafy green salad with slices of avocado.

Dinner: Garlic Bread

Time: 70 minutes

Makes: 10 buns

Serving Size: ½ a bun

Prep Time: 20 minutes

Cook Time: 50 minutes

Nutritional Value (per serving):

Net carbs	*1g*
Fat	*8g*
Protein	*2g*

Calories	91

Ingredients for the bread:

- 1 ¼ cup almond flour
- 5 tbsp psyllium husk powder
- 2 tsp baking powder
- 1 tsp sea salt
- 1 cup water
- 2 tsp white wine vinegar
- 3 egg whites

Ingredients for the garlic butter:

- 4 oz butter (room temperature)
- 1 clove garlic, minced
- 2 tbsp fresh parsley, finely chopped
- ½ tsp salt

Directions:

1. While the oven is preheating to 350°F, line a baking tray with parchment paper. Use a mixing bowl to combine the almond flour, ground psyllium husk powder, baking powder, and sea salt.
2. Add a cup of water to a pot and bring it to a boil. Introduce the hot water, egg whites, and vinegar to the dry ingredients and blend with a mixer. Be careful not to over-mix the ingredients. It should resemble the texture of playdough.
3. Keep your hands wet when you shape the dough into 10 pieces. Roll each piece into the shape of a hot dog bun and put them on the lined baking tray. Make sure you leave enough space between each piece as they will swell when baking.
4. Pop them in the oven for 40 to 50 minutes.

5. While your bread is baking, start preparing the garlic butter by combining all the garlic butter ingredients in a bowl. Cover the butter and place it in the fridge.
6. Remove the bread from the oven and allow it to cool down for a few minutes.
7. Slice the buns in half and use the garlic butter as a scrumptious spread! Turn the oven up to 425°F, and place your garlic buns in the oven for 10 to 15 minutes to allow the butter to seep into the bread. They'll turn a beautiful golden color once they're ready.

Day 5

Breakfast (Optional): Cranberry and Kale Salad

Time: 20 minutes

Makes: 6 servings

Prep Time: 10 minutes

Cook Time: 10 minutes

Nutritional Value (per serving):

Net carbs	*2g*
Fat	*13g*
Protein	*1g*

Calories	*127*

Ingredients:

- 2 cups kale, chopped
- ⅛ tsp salt
- 3 tbsp olive oil
- 3 tbsp mayonnaise
- 3 tbsp orange juice
- 1 tbsp orange zest
- ½ red onion, sliced
- ⅓ cup fresh cranberries or pomegranate seeds
- ⅓ oz pumpkin seeds, roasted and salted

Directions:

1. In a bowl, combine the salt, kale, and 1 tbsp of olive oil. Use your hands to gently rub the salt and olive oil into the kale and place it aside.
2. Combine the remainder of the olive oil with mayonnaise, orange juice, and orange zest in a smaller bowl until it develops a velvety texture.
3. Before serving (5 to 10 minutes), combine the kale combination with the pumpkin seeds, cranberries, and onions together. Stir the homemade dressing that you made through your salad and enjoy!
4. You can substitute the orange juice and zest with lemon juice and balsamic vinegar. Change it up a little by using toasted pecan nuts instead of pumpkin seeds or ditch the kale and use spinach instead.

Lunch: Tortilla Pizzas

Time: 50 minutes

Makes: 4 servings

Serving Size: 1 pizza

Prep Time: 30 minutes

Cook Time: 20 minutes

Nutritional Value (per serving):

Net carbs	*5g*
Fat	*30g*
Protein	*21g*
Calories	*377*

Ingredients for the tortillas:
- 2 large eggs
- 2 large egg whites
- 6 oz cream cheese (room temperature)
- ¼ tsp salt
- 1 tsp ground psyllium husk powder
- 1 tbsp coconut flour

Ingredients for the topping:
- ½ cup unsweetened tomato sauce (divided)
- 2 cups shredded mozzarella cheese
- 2 tsp dried basil or dried oregano

Directions for the tortillas:

1. While you're waiting for the oven to preheat to 400°F, line two baking trays with parchment paper and place them to the side.
2. Combine the eggs and the egg whites in a bowl using an electric mixer until they start to fluff up. Fold in the cream cheese until a batter forms.
3. Combine the coconut flour, psyllium husk, and salt in a small bowl. Add a spoon of this dry combination to your batter and beat the batter. Repeat this step until the batter thickens and allow it to rest for a few minutes.
4. Spread the batter on the parchment paper, forming four thin circles (¼ inch thick). Place the baking tray in the oven for 15 minutes, remove, and allow them to cool down.

Directions for building your pizzas:

1. Turn up the oven's temperature to 450°F.
2. Smear the tomato sauce as a base on each baked tortilla and add cheese and basil (or oregano).
3. Pop your pizzas in the oven for 5 minutes to melt the cheese, serve, and enjoy!

Dinner: Grilled Portobello "Steaks"

Time: 20 minutes

Makes: 2 servings

Prep Time: 10 minutes

Cook Time: 10 minutes

Nutritional Value (per serving):

Net carbs	12g
Fat	56g
Protein	7g
Calories	583

Ingredients for the portobello steaks:

- 4 portobello mushrooms
- 2 tbsp olive oil
- 2 tsp sea salt
- 1 tsp pepper

Ingredients for the avocado chimichurri:

- 1 fresh jalapeño
- 2 cloves garlic
- 1 shallot
- 1 avocado
- 1 lemon or lime, juiced
- 2 tbsp fresh parsley
- ½ tsp sea salt
- ½ tsp pepper
- 4 tbsp olive oil

Directions:

1. Preheat your grill on medium-low heat covered. While you're waiting for the grill to warm up, clean the mushrooms and cut off the stems. Paint both sides of the mushrooms with olive oil and dust them with salt and pepper as desired.

2. Put your mushrooms stem-side down on the grill and cook them for 5 minutes. Flip them and paint the top side with more olive oil.
3. Chop up your jalapeños (remove the seeds if you don't want a dish that's too spicy), garlic, and shallots. Slice your avocado in half and de-stone it before removing the flesh to cut into pieces.
4. In a food processor, combine the jalapeños, garlic, shallots, and avocado. Add your lemon juice, olive oil, and parsley to the combination and sprinkle it with salt and pepper to taste. Beat the combination until it becomes chunky.
5. Get your mushrooms off the grill and place them on a plate (stem-side down). Top them with your chimichurri mixture and dust with salt to taste.
6. You can fry your mushrooms in a pan over medium-high heat for 5 to 7 minutes per side instead of using a grill.

Day 6

Breakfast (Optional): Crispy Sesame Bread

Time: 1 hour and 3 minutes

Makes: 10 servings

Serving Size: 3

Prep Time: 3 minutes

Cook Time: 1 hour

Nutritional Value (per serving):

Net carbs	3g
Fat	15g
Protein	6g
Calories	183

Ingredients:

- 1 ¼ cup sesame seeds
- ½ cup sunflower seeds
- ½ cup shredded cheddar cheese
- 1 tbsp ground psyllium husk powder
- ½ cup water
- 2 eggs
- ¼ tsp salt

Directions:

1. While you're waiting for the oven to preheat to 350°F, start by lining a rectangular baking tray with parchment paper.
2. Combine all of the ingredients in a mixing bowl and mix well.
3. Spread the mixture on the parchment paper (approximately ⅛ of an inch thick) and dust the top with some sea salt.
4. Place the baking tray in the oven for 20 minutes. Remove the tray from the oven and slice the crispy bread into squares.
5. Reduce the heat to 275°F and put the baking tray back into the oven for 30 to 40 minutes.
6. To make sure that they are dry, switch off the oven and leave the oven door slightly ajar (do not remove the crispy bread yet). Once the oven has cooled down completely, remove the tray and serve.

Lunch: Goat Cheese Salad With Balsamic Vinegar

Time: 15 minutes

Makes: 2 servings

Prep Time: 5 minutes

Cook Time: 10 minutes

Nutritional Value (per serving):

Net carbs	*3g*
Fat	*73g*
Protein	*37g*
Calories	*826*

Ingredients:

- 10 oz goat cheese
- ¼ cup pumpkin seeds
- 2 oz butter
- 1 tbsp balsamic vinegar
- 3 oz baby spinach

Directions:

1. While the oven is preheating to 400°F, grease a baking tray or dish and put the goat cheese in it. Pop it in the oven for 10 minutes.
2. While the goat cheese is in the oven, cook the pumpkin seeds in a pan on high heat until they start to burst open.

3. Place butter in the pan, turn the heat down and allow it to slowly cook until the pumpkin seeds start to give off a nutty scent.
4. Pour in the balsamic vinegar and allow it to boil for a few minutes. Switch off the stove.
5. Place your baby spinach leaves on a plate and top them with the baked cheese. Drizzle the balsamic butter mixture over your salad before serving.

Dinner: Vegetarian Tapas

Time: 50 minutes

Makes: 8 servings

Prep Time: 15 minutes

Cook Time: 35 minutes

Nutritional Value (per serving):

Net carbs	3g
Fat	9g
Protein	5g
Calories	119

Ingredients:
- 1 large eggplant
- 1 large zucchini
- 2 flame-roasted peppers
- 1 clove garlic, crushed

- 3 tbsp olive oil
- 10 oz ricotta cheese
- ½ cup Parmesan cheese, finely grated
- 3 sun-dried tomatoes, chopped
- 1 tbsp lemon zest
- 5 basil leaves
- ½ cup parsley, chopped
- ½ tsp paprika

Directions:

1. Slice the eggplant and zucchini thinly (you should have 8 slices of each). Cut off the ends of the peppers and rid them of seeds before cutting them into quarters.
2. Combine the garlic and olive oil in a bowl and set it aside.
3. Heat a grill pan on medium heat. Paint the veggie slices with your garlic and olive oil combination and put them in the pan to cook for 2 to 3 minutes on each side until charred.
4. Combine the sun-dried tomatoes, lemon zest, and cheeses in a bowl and sprinkle with salt and pepper as desired.
5. Lay out the charred eggplant slices and top them with zucchini, a strip of pepper, and a basil leaf. Top each with a dollop of cheese mixture and roll them up. Put a cocktail stick through them to keep them in place. Dust your rolls lightly with paprika and garnish them with chopped parsley before serving.

Day 7

Breakfast (Optional): Avocado Smoothie

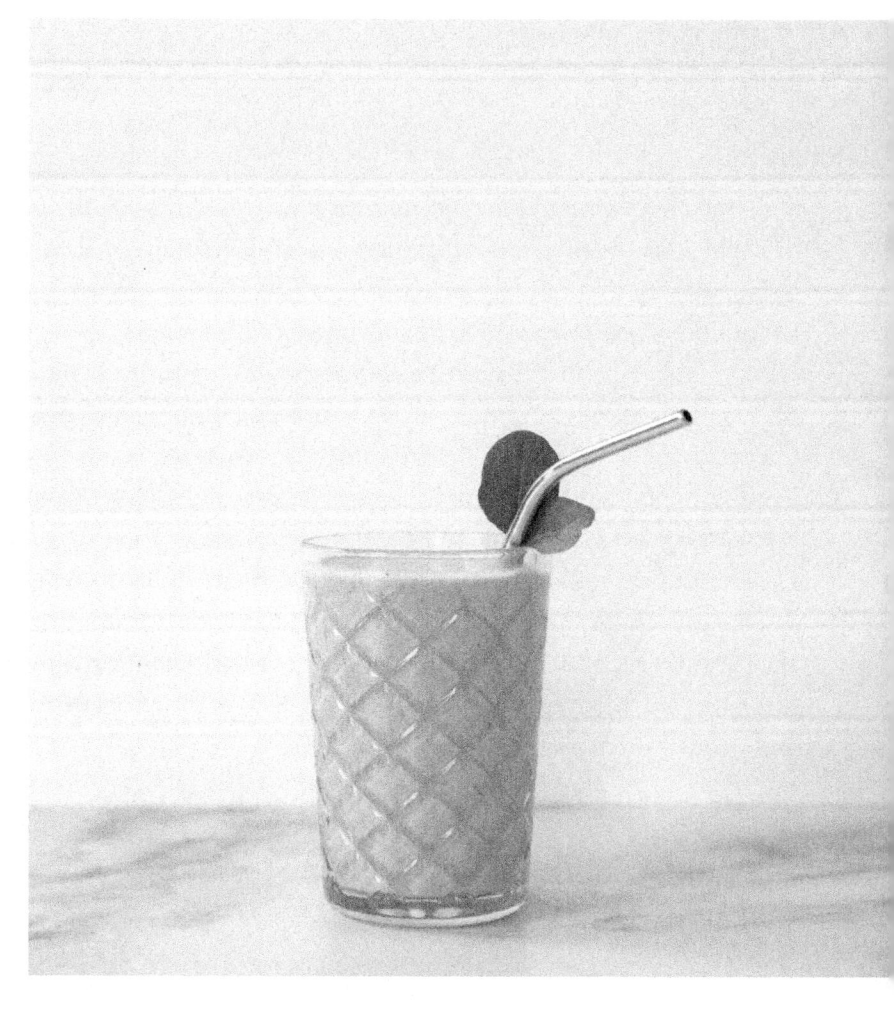

Time: 5 minutes

Makes: 2 servings

Prep Time: 5 minutes

Nutritional Value (per serving):

Net carbs	3g
Fat	6g
Protein	2g
Calories	71

Ingredients:

- ½ large avocado
- 1 ½ cups coconut milk
- 1 tsp vanilla extract
- 2 tbsp stevia
- ⅛ tsp salt
- A scoop of protein powder (optional)

Directions:

1. Peel the avocado and remove the stone.
2. Using a blender, combine all the ingredients until they form a velvety texture and serve.

Lunch: Stuffed Zucchini Skins

Time: 30 minutes

Makes: 6 servings

Prep Time: 10 minutes

Cook Time: 20 minutes

Nutritional Value (per serving):

Net carbs	3g
Fat	8g
Protein	6g
Calories	108

Ingredients:

- 3 large zucchinis, halved and seeds removed
- 1 ½ tsp salt
- 3 whole cremini mushrooms, diced
- 1 tsp olive oil
- 2 tsp smoked paprika
- 1 tbsp Worcestershire sauce
- 2 oz Pepper Jack cheese, shredded
- 2 oz cheddar cheese, shredded
- 3 tbsp sour cream
- 2 tbsp chives, chopped

Directions:

1. While the oven is preheating to 375°F, dust the zucchini skins with salt and set them aside to allow the moisture to seep out, and use a kitchen towel to pat them dry.
2. Combine the mushrooms with olive oil, smoked paprika, salt, and Worcestershire sauce.
3. Scoop the mushroom mixture into the hollowed-out zucchini skins. Place them on a baking tray and pop them in the oven for 8 to 10 minutes or until you can hear them sizzling.
4. Take the baking tray out of the oven to top the mushroom-stuffed zucchinis with Pepper Jack cheese and cheddar cheese

and place them back into the oven for an additional 5 to 10 minutes (until the cheese bubbles).
5. Before serving, top each zucchini with a dollop of sour cream and a sprinkle of chives.

Dinner: Cheesy Ratatouille

Time: 1 hour and 35 minutes

Makes: 8 servings

Prep Time: 20 minutes

Cook Time: 1 hour and 15 minutes

Nutritional Value (per serving):

Net carbs	9g
Fat	20g
Protein	7g
Calories	257

Ingredients for the ratatouille:
- ¼ cup olive oil
- 2 small red onions, thinly sliced
- 2 cloves garlic, minced
- 2 large eggplants, diced
- 1 small red bell pepper, thinly sliced
- 1 tsp smoked paprika
- 2 ½ tbsp coconut aminos
- 2 cups tomato sauce

- 3 ½ oz soft goat cheese
- 2 small zucchinis, thinly sliced

Ingredients for the cheese sauce:

- ¼ cup heavy cream
- 2 tbsp butter
- ¼ cup cream cheese
- ½ cup grated cheddar cheese
- Salt to taste

Directions:

1. In a pan, melt the butter and introduce the cream cheese and cream. Stir well. Once everything is stirred, sprinkle the grated cheese into the mixture and combine until a thick sauce begins to develop. Set the sauce aside.
2. While the oven is preheating to 450°F, fry the onions and garlic in olive oil over medium heat until the onions soften. Then, add your diced eggplant, chopped bell pepper, and an additional tbsp of olive oil and fry for another 5 minutes.
3. Add your coconut aminos, spice it up with some paprika, and throw in the tomato sauce. Combine everything well and allow it to boil slowly for 5 minutes. Remove the pan from the heat and set it aside.
4. Scoop your ratatouille base into an ovenproof dish, pour the cheese sauce over the base, and even it out.
5. Cover the top of your dish with the sliced zucchini and crumble the goat cheese over the laid-out zucchini layer.
6. Add a drizzle of olive oil and a dash of salt to top it off and place the dish in the oven to cook for 20 to 30 minutes. The zucchini will start to develop a honey-brown color.
7. Remove the dish from the oven and allow it to cool down before serving it with a dash of fresh or dried herbs. You can store this dish in an airtight container for up to one week.

Day 8

Breakfast (Optional): Spinach and Feta Crustless Quiche

Time: 55 minutes

Makes: 8 servings

Serving size: 1 slice

Prep Time: 10 minutes

Cook Time: 45 minutes

Nutritional Value (per serving):

Net carbs	3g
Fat	20g
Protein	9g
Calories	234

Ingredients:
- 1 tbsp butter
- 4 large eggs
- 1 cup heavy whipping cream
- ⅔ cup crumbled feta cheese
- ¼ cup Parmesan cheese, finely grated
- 1 cup fresh spinach, chopped
- ½ cup mozzarella, grated

- A pinch of salt and pepper
- 1 tsp onion powder
- ½ tsp garlic powder

Directions:

1. While the oven is preheating to 350°F, grease a baking tray (8 inches) with butter.
2. Beat the eggs and cream in a bowl. Add the onion powder garlic powder, and salt and pepper as desired as well as the Parmesan and half of the grated mozzarella cheese. Set your mixture aside.
3. Sprinkle the spinach evenly over the base of your greased baking tray and add the crumbled feta on top of the layer of spinach. Pour the egg combination over the spinach and feta and top it off with the remaining mozzarella.
4. Pop it in the oven for 45 minutes or until the mixture looks like it has set.
5. Allow it to cool for a few minutes before serving.

Lunch: Cured and Marinated Halloumi Bites

Time: 30 minutes

Makes: 2 servings

Serving size: 4 Halloumi sticks

Prep Time: 15 minutes

Cook Time: 15 minutes

Nutritional Value (per serving):

Net carbs	3g
Fat	55g
Protein	25g
Calories	605

Ingredients:

- 9 oz Halloumi cheese
- 2 tsp curry spice mix
- 2 tbsp olive oil
- 1 tbsp ghee
- Fresh herbs (cilantro) to serve

Directions:

1. Cut the Halloumi into 8 ½-inch slices.
2. Combine the spice with olive oil to form a puree. Brush the Halloumi on all sides with your spicy olive oil puree.
3. Put them in the fridge to develop flavor for a minimum of 15 minutes (a few hours is recommended, but if you're pressed for time, 15 minutes will suffice).
4. In a frying pan, melt the ghee over medium heat. Place the Halloumi slices in the pan and fry them for 3 to 4 minutes on each side or until they turn a beautiful tanned color.
5. Remove them from the pan and serve immediately. Halloumi is best served warm. You can store it in the fridge for up to three days and simply reheat it to eat.

Dinner: Roasted Onion and Cauliflower Soup

Time: 1 hour

Makes: 6 servings

Serving size: 1 cup

Prep Time: 10 minutes

Cook Time: 50 minutes

Nutritional Value (per serving):

Net carbs	7g
Fat	23g
Protein	9g
Calories	274

Ingredients:

- 2 large brown onions
- ½ head cauliflower
- 4 cloves garlic, still in the skin
- 4 tbsp ghee
- ½ tbsp sea salt
- ¼ tsp ground pepper
- 4 cups vegetable stock
- 1 cup water
- 1 cup grated cheese (your choice)

Directions:

1. While the oven is preheating to 375°F, break the cauliflower into florets and slice the onions. Mix them together in a baking tray with the whole garlic cloves, olive oil, and a dash of salt and pepper.
2. Put the tray with the vegetables in the oven to cook for 45 minutes, stirring it halfway through to prevent the vegetables from sticking to the tray.
3. Once the vegetables have finished roasting, remove the tray from the oven and pick out the whole cloves of garlic. Pour the roasted vegetables into a pot with the vegetable stock and water. Squeeze the garlic out of their skins into the pot. Bring the vegetable mix to a slow boil for 10 minutes.
4. Remove the pot from the stove and serve your delicious onion soup with a topping of grated cheese.

Day 9

Breakfast (Optional): Pancake Cereal

Time: 25 minutes

Makes: 4 servings

Serving size: Approximately 1 cup

Prep Time: 15 minutes

Cook Time: 10 minutes

Nutritional Value (per serving):

Net carbs	4g
Fat	38g
Protein	12g
Calories	406

Ingredients:

- 4 large eggs
- ¼ cup melted ghee
- 1 cup almond flour
- 4 tbsp granulated erythritol
- ½ tsp cinnamon
- 2 tsp baking powder
- 2 tbsp ghee for cooking
- Whipped cream and berries of choice (optional)

Directions:

1. Beat the eggs and ghee together in a bowl.
2. In a large bowl, mix the cinnamon, sweetener, almond flour, and baking powder together before adding the eggs and ghee and stir well until it forms a velvety texture.
3. Transfer the batter into a squeezy bottle and set aside.
4. Grease a nonstick pan and place it on medium-high heat. Once the pan is warm, reduce the temperature. Squeeze small dollops of batter into the pan (about 1 inch in size) and allow it to fry for approximately 2 minutes. Once bubbles form on the top of the small pancakes, flip them and cook them for another 2 minutes. Repeat until you've finished frying all the batter. Continue to grease the pan as needed.

5. You can serve your pancake cereal with whipped cream, nuts, or Greek yogurt. Feel free to get creative and add a splash of berries or cinnamon for a burst of flavor.

Lunch: Easy Warm Egg Salad

Time: 50 minutes

Makes: 3 servings

Prep Time: 15 minutes

Cook Time: 35 minutes

Nutritional Value (per serving):

Net carbs	*9g*
Fat	*36g*
Protein	*14g*
Calories	*412*

Ingredients for the salad:
- 3 large eggs, hard-boiled
- ½ medium head cauliflower
- 1 medium leek (white and light green parts only)
- 1 tbsp olive oil

Ingredients for the lemony pesto salad dressing:
- ¼ cup green pesto
- 3 tbsp lemon juice
- 1 ½ tbsp mayonnaise

- ¼ tsp salt

Ingredients for the toppings:
- 2 tbsp pepitas
- 2 tbsp capers
- ⅓ cup crumbled feta cheese
- A handful of herbs (your choice)

Directions:
1. While the oven is preheating to 355°F, break the cauliflower into small florets and drizzle the florets with olive oil and a dash of salt. Place them on an oven tray and cook them in the oven for 15 minutes.
2. Remove the tray from the oven, and combine the leeks with the cauliflower. Pop the tray back into the oven to cook for an additional 15 to 20 minutes. Once cooked, remove them from the oven and set aside to cool down.
3. In a bowl, combine the green pesto, lemon juice, mayonnaise, and salt as desired and stir well.
4. Transfer the slightly cooled vegetables to a serving dish and crumble the eggs all over. Pour the dressing over the vegetables and crumbled eggs.
5. Top off your dish with pepitas, capers, and feta and serve immediately. You're welcome to add a dash of mixed herbs for a pop of green.

Dinner: Curry Bake

Time: 45 minutes

Makes: 4 servings

Prep Time: 10 minutes

Cook Time: 35 minutes

Nutritional Value (per serving):

Net carbs	8g
Fat	30g
Protein	20g
Calories	387

Ingredients:

- 9 oz Halloumi cheese
- 1 small red pepper
- 2 cups button mushrooms
- 1 cup green beans, trimmed
- 3 spring onions
- 1 tbsp curry powder
- ⅛ tsp garlic powder
- 1 tsp masala powder
- ½ cup sour cream
- 3 tbsp ghee
- 1 tbsp water
- ½ tsp salt
- ¼ tsp pepper
- 4 tbsp full-fat yogurt or sour cream to serve with

- Fresh cilantro to serve with

Directions:

1. While you're waiting for the oven to preheat to 400°F, mix all the spices with salt and pepper in a bowl. Make a paste by adding ½ cup of sour cream, ghee, and a tbsp of water to the spices and stirring the mixture well. Don't worry if the combination solidifies.
2. Cut the Halloumi cheese into small cubes and set aside.
3. Cut the tops off the pepper and rid it of seeds before cutting it into cubes. Slice up the green beans and cut the mushrooms in half. Remove the green ends from the spring onions and cut them in half.
4. Combine your vegetables and cubes of Halloumi cheese with the curry paste and mix it thoroughly.
5. Grease a baking tray with the remainder of the ghee and spread the curry vegetable and Halloumi mixture evenly in the tray. Pop it in the oven and allow it to cook for 30 to 35 minutes or until the edge of the elements start to tan.
6. Remove the tray from the oven and serve immediately. You can serve this delicious dish with a dollop of cream cheese or full-fat yogurt and a dash of fresh cilantro.

Day 10

Breakfast (Optional): Caprese Paninis

Time: 40 minutes

Makes: 4 servings

Serving Size: 1 panini

Prep Time: 10 minutes

Cook Time: 30 minutes

Nutritional Value (per serving):

Net carbs	*9g*
Fat	*43g*
Protein	*37g*
Calories	*569*

Ingredients for the ciabatta bread:
- 1 ¾ cup shredded and low-moisture mozzarella cheese
- 1 ½ cup almond flour
- 1 heaped tbsp cream cheese
- 2 tsp baking powder
- 1 large egg

Ingredients for the panini filling:

- 16 basil leaves
- 1 Italian tomato, thinly sliced
- 9 oz fresh mozzarella
- Salt and pepper to taste

Directions:

1. While the oven is preheating to 425°F, put the mozzarella and cream cheese in a bowl and heat it in the microwave for 1 minute on high. Remove it to combine. Repeat this every 30 seconds until the cheese has melted and the consistency has become velvety.
2. Combine all the dry ingredients in a mixing bowl. Break in the eggs and pour the mozzarella combination into the mixture. Beat the batter until it becomes a smooth dough.
3. Equally divide the dough into four rectangular shapes and put them on a lined baking tray. Pop them in the oven for 15 to 20 minutes. Set them aside to cool down once they're ready.
4. Turn on your panini press once the buns have cooled down completely. Split the buns open and stuff them with mozzarella, tomato slices, basil leaves, and salt and pepper as desired. Grill them in the panini press until the cheese has melted and the buns have developed a tan color.
5. Serve immediately while they're still warm!

Lunch: Savory Veggie Loaf

Time: 1 hour and 20 minutes

Makes: 12 slices

Serving Size: 1 slice

Prep Time: 15 minutes

Cook Time: 1 hour and 5 minutes

Nutritional Value (per serving):

Net carbs	*4g*
Fat	*15g*
Protein	*7g*
Calories	*175*

Ingredients:

- 1 cup almond flour
- ½ cup mixed seeds
- ⅓ cup coconut flour
- 2 tbsp psyllium husk powder
- 1 large zucchini, grated
- 1 small carrot, grated
- 1 cup pumpkin, grated
- 4 extra large eggs (or 5 medium eggs)
- ¼ cup coconut oil
- 1 tbsp smoked paprika
- 2 tsp ground cumin
- 2 tbsp baking powder

- 2 tbsp salt
- 2 tbsp mixed seeds to garnish

Directions:

1. While the oven is preheating to 340°F, mix the baking powder, seeds, psyllium, almond flour, coconut flour, spices, and salt together in a bowl.
2. In a different bowl, combine the ghee and eggs with the grated vegetables. Add the dry ingredients to the vegetables and stir. The combination will look dry. Pour the mixture into a bread pan and sprinkle it with ½ cup of mixed seeds.
3. Pop the bread pan into the oven and allow it to cook for 55 to 70 minutes or until a skewer comes out dry. Remove the bread from the oven and allow it to cool down for at least 30 minutes before removing it from the pan and placing it on a cooling rack.
4. You can store it in an airtight container in the fridge for up to 5 days for an easy breakfast or top it with eggs for a light dinner.

Dinner: Mushroom and Ricotta Galette

Time: 50 minutes

Makes: 6 servings

Prep Time: 25 minutes

Cook Time: 25 minutes

Nutritional Value (per serving):

Net carbs	7g
Fat	33g
Protein	21g
Calories	406

Ingredients for the filling:
- 1 clove garlic, minced
- 1 small onion, grated
- 2 ½ cups mixed mushrooms, thickly sliced
- 2 tbsp fresh thyme
- 7 large eggs
- 3 tbsp butter (divided)
- 1 cup ricotta cheese (divided)
- ½ cup Gouda cheese, grated
- 1 tbsp olive oil

Ingredients for the dough:
- 1 cup almond flour
- 1 ½ cup mozzarella cheese, grated
- 1 heaped tbsp cream cheese
- 1 large egg
- 1 tsp onion powder
- ½ tsp garlic powder
- 1 tsp Italian seasoning

Directions:
1. Melt half the butter in a pan and add the sliced mushrooms to fry until they're crispy.

2. While the mushrooms are frying, melt the remainder of the butter in a small saucepan and add the chopped onion and garlic to saute until the onions turn translucent.
3. Add the ricotta, Gouda, thyme leaves, eggs, and saucepan mixture to a bowl and mix well until you're left with a lovely creamy combination. Set it aside.
4. While the oven is preheating to 425°F, melt the mozzarella and cream cheese in the microwave on high for 1 minute. Remove it and beat well before placing it back into the microwave for an additional 30 seconds. Stir the almond flour, eggs, and spices into the melted cheese until a velvety smooth dough forms.
5. Place the dough between sheets of parchment paper and roll it out thinly into a rough circle. Set your dough aside.
6. Scoop the ricotta mixture onto the middle of the dough and spread it so that you're left with 1-inch borders. Sprinkle the mushrooms over the ricotta mixture evenly and fold the sides of the dough inward. You should still be able to see the ricotta and mushrooms when the edges have been folded inward.
7. Pop it in the oven for 25 minutes. Before serving, add a drizzle of olive oil over your galette and extra fresh thyme if desired.

Day 11

Breakfast (Optional): English Veggie Bowl

Time: 35 minutes

Makes: 1 serving

Prep Time: 15 minutes

Cook Time: 20 minutes

Nutritional Value (per serving):

Net carbs	*10g*
Fat	*60g*
Protein	*16g*
Calories	*662*

Ingredients:

- 1 small bell pepper, sliced and de-seeded
- 2 tsp ghee (divided)
- A pinch of salt
- 1 tsp pumpkin seeds
- 1 tsp sunflower seeds
- 1 tsp flaxseed
- 1 tbsp olive oil
- ¾ cup shredded kale or spinach
- ⅓ cup sliced white mushrooms
- 3 slices Halloumi cheese

- 1 tbsp marinara sauce
- A few basil leaves

Ingredients for the smashed avocado:

- ½ small avocado
- 1 tsp fresh lime juice
- 1 tsp olive oil
- A pinch of salt and pepper
- ⅛ tsp chili flakes

Directions:

1. While the oven is preheating to 400°F, put the sliced bell pepper on a baking tray and sprinkle it with olive oil and a pinch of salt. Place the tray in the oven for 25 minutes or until the bell pepper has softened up.
2. On another baking tray, spread the seeds and place the tray in the oven for approximately 4 minutes. Remove them from the oven to allow them to cool down.
3. In a nonstick pan, melt the butter over medium heat and cook the mushrooms for 2 minutes. Then, add the kale or spinach and allow it to cook for an additional 2 minutes.
4. In a different pan, fry the Halloumi in a tsp of olive oil for 2 minutes on each side.
5. In a bowl, press the avocado with a fork before stirring in the chili flakes, lime, salt and pepper, and olive oil.
6. Put the mushrooms and kale (or spinach) mixture in a bowl and top it with the toasted seeds and peppers. Put some Halloumi on the side, and top off your dish with your smashed avocado, marinara sauce, and a dash of fresh basil. This dish is best served fresh.

Lunch: Jalapeño Cheese Bread

Time: 20 minutes

Makes: 8 servings

Prep Time: 5 minutes

Cook Time: 15 minutes

Nutritional Value (per serving):

Net carbs	2g
Fat	6g
Protein	6g
Calories	92

Ingredients:

- 4 large eggs
- 2 heaped tbsp full-fat Greek yogurt
- ⅓ cup coconut flour
- 2 tbsp whole psyllium husk
- ½ tsp sea salt
- 1 tsp baking powder
- ½ cup shredded cheddar cheese (divided)
- ¼ diced, pickled jalapeño
- A few slices of fresh jalapeño for topping
- Serve with ranch dressing (optional)

Directions:
1. While the oven is preheating to 375°F, line a baking tray with parchment paper.
2. In a bowl, beat the eggs and Greek yogurt together. Add the baking powder, salt, psyllium husk, and coconut flour and stir in through before adding half of the shredded cheddar cheese. Lastly, mix the diced jalapeño with the mixture until a rough dough forms.
3. Create a circle and press down on the dough until it is about 1 inch thick. Sprinkle cheese over the top and additional jalapeños if desired.
4. Pop your loaf into the oven for 15 minutes until it develops a tanned color and puffs up.
5. Slice the bread into eight squares before serving. You can serve this bread warm or cold with a thin spread of ranch dressing.

Dinner: Roasted "Potatoes" With Garlic and Feta

Time: 40 minutes

Makes: 6 servings

Prep Time: 5 minutes

Cook Time: 35 minutes

Nutritional Value (per serving):

Net carbs	7g
Fat	15g
Protein	6g
Calories	186

Ingredients:

- 1 large celeriac, peeled
- 1 small cauliflower
- 4 cloves garlic
- 4 tbsp olive oil or melted butter
- 2 tsp dried oregano
- 3 tbsp fresh rosemary
- 1 tsp fresh thyme
- 1 cup crumbled feta cheese
- ½ tsp sea salt
- Fresh oregano or herbs of choice for garnish

Directions:

1. While the oven is preheating to 410°F, slice the celeriac into 1-inch cubes and break the cauliflower into small florets. Peel and chop the garlic finely.
2. In a baking tray, spread the celeriac, garlic, and cauliflower out evenly. Top them with herbs and olive oil or melted butter and sprinkle with salt. Combine the elements well and place them in the oven for 30 to 35 minutes or until the edges have started tanning.

3. Serve it with a topping of oregano and crumbled feta for a delicious yet light dinner or a side dish. You're welcome to double the serving for a fully satisfying meal.

Day 12

Breakfast (Optional): Caprese Omelet

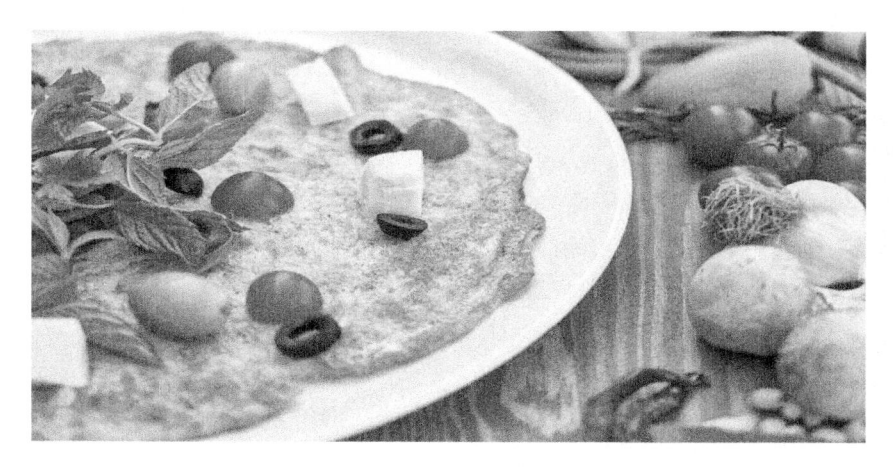

Time: 15 minutes

Makes: 1 serving

Prep Time: 10 minutes

Cook Time: 5 minutes

Nutritional Value (per serving):

Net carbs	4g
Fat	43g
Protein	30g
Calories	533

Ingredients:

- 3 large eggs
- 1 tbsp ghee
- ¾ cup cherry tomatoes halved
- 2 slices fresh mozzarella
- 3 to 6 basil leaves, chopped
- 1 heaped tbsp grated Parmesan
- 1 tbsp pesto
- Salt and pepper to taste
- 1 tsp balsamic vinegar to drizzle on top

Directions:

1. Beat the eggs and 1 tbsp of water in a mixing bowl. Melt the ghee in a nonstick pan over low heat. Pour the mixture into the pan and continuously tilt the pan so that the eggs cook evenly. When the top of the eggs is no longer runny, top one side with mozzarella, Parmesan, basil, and half of the tomatoes.
2. Fold the other half over to cover the ingredients and put it on a plate. Top off your omelet with pesto and the remainder of the tomatoes.
3. If desired, add a drizzle of balsamic vinegar over the omelet. Serve immediately.

Lunch: Roasted Pumpkin Salad

Time: 1 hour

Makes: 4 servings

Prep Time: 10 minutes

Cook Time: 50 minutes

Nutritional Value (per serving):

Net carbs	*7g*
Fat	*27g*
Protein	*10g*
Calories	*299*

Ingredients:
- 11 oz pumpkin, cubed
- 1 cup crumbled feta
- 2 oz arugula
- 4 tbsp olive oil
- 1 tbsp coconut aminos
- 5 tbsp pepitas
- Salt and pepper as desired

Directions:
1. While the oven is preheating to 425°F, spread out the pumpkin on a baking tray and add a dash of olive oil and coconut aminos. Sprinkle the pumpkin with salt and pepper to taste and

pop it in the oven for 20 to 30 minutes. Remove the pumpkin from the oven to allow it to cool down.
2. Lay the arugula out in a bowl and sprinkle the pumpkin and crumbled feta over it. Top it off with pepitas and a drizzle of olive oil before serving.

Dinner: Baked Italian Mushrooms

Time: 30 minutes

Makes: 4 servings

Prep Time: 10 minutes

Cook Time: 20 minutes

Nutritional Value (per serving):

Net carbs	*6g*
Fat	*16g*
Protein	*14g*
Calories	*231*

Ingredients:

- 4 portobello mushrooms
- 1 large can unsweetened tomatoes
- 1 ⅓ cups Parmesan cheese
- 2 tbsp ghee
- 2 tbsp fresh basil
- 1 tbsp fresh parsley
- 1 tsp dried oregano

- Salt and pepper to taste

Directions:

1. While you're waiting for the oven to preheat to 425°F, prepare the mushrooms by cleaning and slicing them.
2. Melt the ghee in a nonstick pan over medium heat and fry the mushrooms for 5 minutes. Sprinkle them with salt and pepper as desired.
3. Remove them from the heat and transfer them to a baking dish.
4. Wash and chop the herbs finely before adding them to a bowl with the canned tomatoes. Season with salt and pepper to taste and stir.
5. Pour the mixture over the mushrooms, sprinkle it with Parmesan cheese, and place it in the oven to cook for 20 to 25 minutes.
6. When your mushrooms are ready, remove them from the oven and allow them to cool down for a few minutes before serving.

Chapter 6:

A 7-Day Meal Plan With Recipes for Vegans

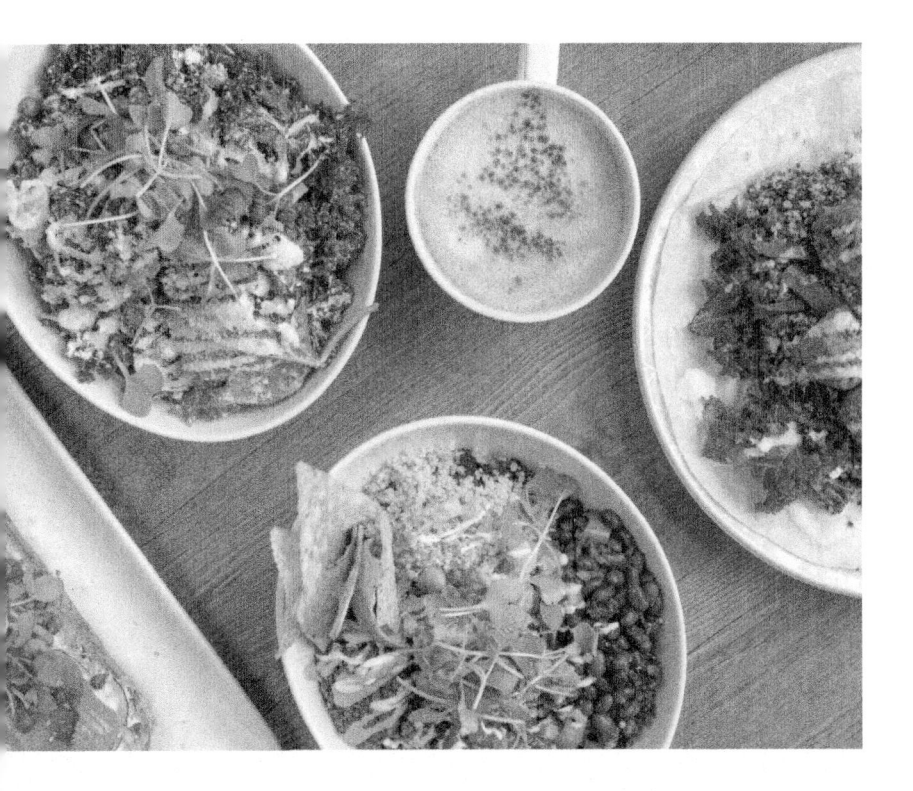

The following meal plan is an example of what a vegan-friendly keto diet should look like. Vegans can consider some meals from the vegetarian meal plan and substitute dairy products with vegan-friendly products. These meals are wholesome and sure to help you shed a few extra pounds and leave you feeling energetic!

The breakfasts are optional for those who want to fast and follow the keto diet. Besides, not everyone is hungry first thing in the morning. For those people, see this as an opportunity to try the breakfast meals for lunch. Feel free to change the meal plan according to your needs. You can store most of these meals to enjoy again the next day!

Day 1

Breakfast (Optional): Grilled Harissa Eggplant

Time: 50 minutes

Makes: 4 servings

Serving Size: ½ of an eggplant

Prep Time: 10 minutes

Cook Time: 40 minutes

Nutritional Value (per serving):

Net carbs	*8g*
Fat	*24g*
Protein	*5g*
Calories	*281*

Ingredients:
- 2 large eggplants, halved
- 4 tbsp avocado oil

- Salt and pepper to taste
- ½ cup tahini dressing
- 1 tsp harissa spice mix (or more to taste)
- 1 tbsp parsley, chopped

Directions:

1. While the oven is preheating to 455°F, cut a crisscross pattern into the skins of your eggplant halves. Generously paint the crisscrossed skin with avocado oil and sprinkle with salt and pepper to taste.
2. Put the eggplants on a baking tray (flesh-side up) and pop them into the oven for 30 to 40 minutes or until the flesh has developed a tanned color.
3. After you've removed the eggplants from the oven, allow them to cool down for at least 5 minutes.
4. Before serving, lightly dress each eggplant half with 2 tbsp of tahini dressing and sprinkle them with chopped parsley.

Lunch: The Immune Booster Soup

Time: 30 minutes

Makes: 6 servings

Serving Size: 1 cup

Prep Time: 15 minutes

Cook Time: 15 minutes

Nutritional Value (per serving):

Net carbs	*8g*
Fat	*25g*
Protein	*15g*
Calories	*312*

Ingredients:

- 2 tbsp coconut oil
- 1 lb fresh broccoli, broken into florets
- 9 oz spinach
- 9 oz fresh kale, chopped finely
- 3 stalks celery, trimmed
- 2 cloves garlic, minced
- 2 tbsp ginger, grated
- 1 can full-fat coconut milk
- 3 cups vegetable stock
- 1 tsp ground turmeric
- 1 cup parsley, chopped (divided)
- Salt and pepper to taste
- 6 tbsp coconut yogurt
- 6 tbsp toasted hemp seeds or coconut seeds
- Chili flakes to taste

Directions:

1. Make sure that all of the moisture has been squeezed out of the spinach and kale.
2. Using a big pot, combine the coconut oil, celery, and garlic and allow it to fry until the celery has softened up. Then, add the grated ginger and allow the ingredients to fry for an additional

minute. Stir in the broccoli florets, spinach, kale, coconut milk, half of the parsley, and vegetable stock. When the mixture starts boiling, reduce the heat and allow it to boil slowly for 10 to 20 minutes. The broccoli should be easy to pierce with a fork.
3. Add the elements of the pot to a blender or a food processor and blend it until it develops a velvety soup texture.
4. Before serving, stir in the coconut yogurt and top off your soup with roasted hemp or coconut seeds and a dash of chili flakes.

Dinner: Superfood Salad Bowl

Time: 25 minutes

Makes: 4 servings

Serving Size: 2 cups

Prep Time: 10 minutes

Cook Time: 15 minutes

Nutritional Value (per serving):

Net carbs	*5g*
Fat	*30g*
Protein	*6g*
Calories	*313*

Ingredients for the salad:

- 1 bunch asparagus
- 1 medium red bell pepper
- 1 small zucchini
- 2 tbsp olive oil
- ½ tsp sea salt
- 2 cups mixed lettuce leaves
- 2 cups fresh spinach
- ½ cup purple cabbage, finely shredded
- 2 medium stalks celery, diced
- 1 avocado, cubed
- ½ cup parsley
- ¼ cup walnuts, roughly chopped

Ingredients for the vinaigrette:

- 3 tbsp olive oil
- 2 tbsp apple cider vinegar
- 2 tsp Dijon mustard
- 2 tsp sweetener (optional)
- Salt and pepper to taste

Directions:

1. While you're waiting for the oven to preheat to 400°F, prepare the roast vegetables by cutting the ends off of the asparagus deseeding the bell pepper, and cutting the asparagus and the bell pepper into thin strips. Dice the zucchini into small cubes.
2. In a baking tray, combine the sliced vegetables with olive oil and salt. Pop them in the oven for 15 to 18 minutes or until the edges have started to tan. Remove your vegetables from the oven and set them aside to cool down slightly.
3. In a jar, combine the olive oil, apple cider vinegar, Dijon mustard, optional sweetener, and salt and pepper as desired.

Shake the jar to stir the ingredients and you have a simple vinaigrette!
4. In a large bowl, combine all of the ingredients and top it with your homemade vinaigrette.

Day 2

Breakfast (Optional): Strawberry and Rhubarb Smoothie

Time: 5 minutes

Makes: 1 serving

Prep Time: 5 minutes

Nutritional Value (per serving):

Net carbs	7g
Fat	26g
Protein	25g
Calories	369

Ingredients:

- 4 tbsp roasted strawberry and rhubarb jam
- 1 cup unsweetened almond milk
- ¼ cup coconut cream
- ¼ cup collagen powder

Directions:

1. Combine all of the ingredients in a blender and beat until it forms a velvety texture.
2. On a hot summer day, add a few ice cubes to your smoothie. Serve, and enjoy your refreshing, wholesome smoothie!

Lunch: Easy Tomato Salad

Time: 10 minutes

Makes: 4 servings

Prep Time: 5 minutes

Cook Time: 5 minutes

Nutritional Value (per serving):

Net carbs	*5g*
Fat	*7g*
Protein	*2g*
Calories	*108*

Ingredients:

- 3 large tomatoes
- 2 medium yellow onions, sliced
- 1 bunch parsley, chopped
- 1 clove garlic, minced
- 2 tbsp apple cider vinegar
- 2 tbsp olive oil
- 1 tbsp sweetener

- ½ tsp salt
- ¼ tsp black pepper

Directions:

1. Slice the tomatoes into wedges and put them in a salad bowl with your sliced onions and minced garlic.
2. Stir the apple cider vinegar, olive oil, sweetener, and salt and pepper together to make a vinaigrette. Make sure the sweetener has dissolved completely.
3. Drizzle your vinaigrette over your salad and toss everything together. Allow your salad to rest for a few minutes before serving.

Dinner: Asian Spiced Broccoli

Time: 25 minutes

Makes: 6 servings

Prep Time: 5 minutes

Cook Time: 20 minutes

Nutritional Value (per serving):

Net carbs	*6g*
Fat	*10g*
Protein	*4g*
Calories	*138*

Ingredients:

- 2 medium heads broccoli, broken into small florets
- 3 tbsp coconut aminos
- 2 cloves garlic, finely chopped
- ½ tsp ground ginger
- ¼ cup olive oil
- ½ tsp chili flakes
- 1 tbsp sesame seeds
- 2 tsp sweetener (optional)
- 1 tsp toasted sesame oil (optional)

Directions:

1. While the oven is preheating to 400°F, put the broccoli florets in a bowl. In a different bowl, combine the coconut aminos, garlic, ground ginger, olive oil, sesame seeds, sweetener, and sesame oil together. Marinate the broccoli by pouring the mixture over the florets and stirring well.
2. Pour the mixture onto a baking tray and cook it in the oven for 20 minutes. Be sure to keep an eye on it so that it doesn't burn.
3. Remove the broccoli mixture from the oven and sprinkle it with some sesame seeds and chili flakes before serving.

Day 3

Breakfast (Optional): Stuffed Avocado

Time: 15 minutes

Makes: 4 servings

Serving Size: ½ of a stuffed avocado

Prep Time: 10 minutes

Cook Time: 5 minutes

Nutritional Value (per serving):

Net carbs	5g
Fat	32g
Protein	5g
Calories	336

Ingredients:
- 2 tbsp avocado oil
- ½ cup grated cauliflower
- ½ cup crushed walnuts
- 1 tbsp chipotle chili in adobo sauce, minced
- ½ tsp cumin
- ½ tsp salt
- 2 large avocados, halved and de-stoned

Ingredients for the salsa:

- 1 Roma tomato, diced
- 1 jalapeño pepper, minced
- 1 tbsp onions, grated
- 1 tbsp cilantro, chopped finely
- ½ small lime, juiced
- Salt and pepper to taste

Ingredients for the chipotle mayonnaise:

- 2 tbsp vegan mayonnaise
- 1 tbsp adobo sauce

Directions:

1. Make your salsa by mixing the tomato, jalapeño, onion, cilantro, lime juice, and salt and pepper in a bowl and set it aside.
2. Prepare the chipotle mayo by stirring the vegan mayonnaise and adobo sauce together. Set it aside.
3. In a pan, fry the cauliflower, walnuts, chipotle spice, and cumin in the avocado oil over medium heat for 5 minutes. The walnuts will toast, and the cauliflower will soften up.
4. Stuff your avocado halves with the fried cauliflower mixture and top it off with your salsa and chipotle mayonnaise.

Lunch: Minty Zucchini Salad

Time: 5 minutes

Makes: 4 servings

Prep Time: 5 minutes

Nutritional Value (per serving):

Net carbs	4g
Fat	7g
Protein	2g
Calories	88

Ingredients:

- 2 large zucchinis
- 2 tbsp olive oil
- 1 tbsp lemon juice
- Salt and pepper to taste
- 1 tbsp chopped mint
- ¼ tsp chili flakes
- 1 tsp lemon zest

Directions:

1. Slice the zucchini into thin strips using a vegetable peeler and put it in a serving bowl.
2. In a small bowl, stir the mint, olive oil, and lemon juice together well. Then, toss it with the zucchini strips.
3. Garnish your dish with a dash of lemon zest and chili flakes before serving.

Dinner: Spicy Vegetable Curry

Time: 45 minutes

Makes: 6 servings

Prep Time: 25 minutes

Cook Time: 20 minutes

Nutritional Value (per serving):

Net carbs	*11g*
Fat	*26g*
Protein	*6g*
Calories	*310*

Ingredients:
- 2 tbsp coconut oil
- 2 cups vegetable stock
- 1 small yellow onion, chopped
- 2 cloves garlic, minced
- 1 tsp ground coriander
- ½ tsp ground turmeric
- 1 tsp ground cumin
- 1 tsp paprika
- 1 small chili pepper, finely sliced
- 1 cup coconut milk
- 1 ¼ cup chopped tomatoes
- 1 medium red pepper, cubed
- 1 medium zucchini, cubed
- 1 large bunch of chopped kale, stems removed

- 1 eggplant, cubed
- 3 tbsp olive oil
- ½ tsp salt
- ¼ tsp black pepper
- 6 cups cauliflower, grated
- 4 tbsp coconut cream

Directions:

1. While you're waiting for the oven to preheat to 375°F, boil the vegetable stock in a pan over medium-low heat until the stock has reduced by half.
2. Place the cubed eggplant on a baking tray and add a dash of olive oil and salt. Cook them in the oven for 20 minutes to tan and soften up.
3. In a saucepan, fry the onion in coconut oil over medium heat for approximately 3 minutes. Then, add garlic to the pan and allow it to fry for an additional minute. Introduce the pepper and zucchini and allow it to cook for another 3 minutes. Pour the reduced stock into your vegetable mixture and stir in the spices, tomatoes, and chili. Sprinkle with salt and pepper as desired and allow it to simmer on medium-low heat for 10 minutes. Then, pour the coconut milk into the mixture and allow it to cook for an additional 10 minutes. Lastly, add the kale and let it boil for 2 to 3 minutes.
4. Remove the pot from the stove and stir in the remainder of the olive oil and the roasted eggplant.
5. Serve your veggie curry on a bed of cauliflower rice with a dash of coconut cream on top.

Day 4

Breakfast (Optional): Blueberry and Lemon Electrolyte Drink

Time: 1 hour

Makes: 6 servings

Serving Size: 1 cup

Prep Time: 10 minutes

Cook Time: 50 minutes

Nutritional Value (per serving):

Net carbs	*5g*
Fat	*0.3g*
Protein	*0.5g*
Calories	*26*

Ingredients:
- 2 cups fresh blueberries
- 4 cups water
- ¼ cup sweetener
- ½ cup lemon juice
- ¼ tsp sea salt
- 2 tbsp natural calm magnesium supplement
- 1 lemon, sliced (to serve)

- Ice (to serve)

Directions:

1. Bring the blueberries and water to boil in a pan over high heat. Once it boils, reduce the heat to low and cook it covered for 2 to 3 minutes. Take the pan off the stove but keep it covered for 20 minutes.
2. Remove the lid and stir the sweetener in. Run the juice through a sieve into a bowl. Use a spoon to crush the blueberries through the sieve. Get rid of the peels that get left behind and allow the juice to cool down to room temperature.
3. Squeeze the lemon juice into the blueberry juice and add the magnesium and salt. Stir it well until all of the ingredients have dissolved. Pour the remaining water into the mixture.
4. Serve with ice cubes to enjoy a refreshing, healthy drink!

Lunch: Cabbage, Avocado, and Almond Salad

Time: 15 minutes

Makes: 3 servings

Prep Time: 15 minutes

Nutritional Value (per serving):

Net carbs	*6g*
Fat	*36g*
Protein	*8g*
Calories	*389*

Ingredients for the salad:

- 3 cups savoy cabbage, shredded
- 1 medium avocado
- ¼ tsp sea salt
- ¼ tsp ground black pepper
- ½ cup blanched almonds

Ingredients for the dressing:

- 3 tbsp olive oil
- 1 tbsp lemon juice
- ½ tsp Dijon mustard
- 1 tsp coconut aminos
- A pinch of salt and pepper

Directions:

1. While the oven is preheating to 375°F, boil water in a pan and add salt.
2. Cut the cabbage into thin slices and add them to the boiling water to cook for 30 seconds to 1 minute. Drain the cabbage and immediately transfer the cabbage into a bowl of ice-cold water. Remove the cabbage from the ice bath and pat it dry with a kitchen towel.
3. In a baking tray, spread the almonds evenly and toast them in the oven for 6 to 8 minutes. Remove the tray and allow the almonds to cool down.
4. Make your dressing by combining the Dijon mustard, lemon juice, olive oil, coconut aminos, salt, and pepper in a bowl.
5. Chop your avocado into chunks and place them in a mixing bowl with your chopped cabbage and almonds. Lightly stir the dressing into your salad.
6. Serve your salad with a dash of black pepper.

Dinner: Braised Fennel With Lemon

Time: 1 hour and 45 minutes

Makes: 6 servings

Prep Time: 10 minutes

Cook Time: 1 hour and 35 minutes

Nutritional Value (per serving):

Net carbs	7g
Fat	9g
Protein	2g
Calories	128

Ingredients:

- 2 lbs fennel bulbs
- 3 large organic lemons
- ¼ cup olive oil
- Salt to taste

Directions:

1. While the oven is preheating to 375°F, cut the fennel and lemons into wedges. Spread the fennel and lemon wedges evenly on a baking tray and add a dash of olive oil and salt. Cover the tray tightly with aluminum foil. Pop them in the oven for an hour. Remove the tray from the oven, uncover, and put it back into the oven to cook for an additional 20 to 30

minutes or until the edges of the fennel crisp up. Serve and enjoy immediately.

Day 5

Breakfast (Optional): Pumpkin Spice Latte

Time: 5 minutes

Makes: 2 servings

Prep Time: 5 minutes

Nutritional Value (per serving):

Net carbs	5g
Fat	38g
Protein	3g
Calories	353

Ingredients:
- 1 cup coconut milk
- 1 cup freshly brewed regular or decaf coffee
- ¼ cup pumpkin puree
- 1 tsp pumpkin pie spice
- ¼ tsp vanilla bean powder
- ¼ tsp turmeric powder
- ⅛ tsp black pepper

- 2 tbsp MCT oil
- Few drops of sweetener (optional)
- 2 tbsp collagen powder (optional)

Directions:

1. In a pan, bring the coconut oil to boil over medium heat. Pour the hot coconut milk and coffee in a blender with the pumpkin pie spice, pumpkin puree, turmeric powder, black pepper, vanilla powder, and MCT oil. Beat the ingredients until they become foamy.
2. Serve your latte piping hot and enjoy!

Lunch: *Sesame Carrot Falafel*

Time: 50 minutes

Makes: 4 servings (12 falafels)

Serving Size: 3 falafels

Prep Time: 30 minutes

Cook Time: 20 minutes

Nutritional Value (per serving):

Net carbs	*12g*
Fat	*23g*
Protein	*5g*
Calories	*292*

Ingredients:

- 3 cloves garlic
- 5 tbsp olive oil
- 16 oz carrots
- 1 tsp ground cumin
- 1 tsp ground coriander
- 2 tbsp fresh lemon juice
- ⅓ cup coconut flour
- 1 ½ tbsp tahini paste
- 1 small bunch fresh cilantro, stalks removed
- Salt and pepper to taste
- 2 tbsp sesame seeds

Directions:

1. While you're waiting for the oven to preheat to 400°F, place the whole cloves on a baking tray and add a dash of olive oil. Pop them in the oven for 12 minutes and remove from the oven. Allow the cloves to cool down for a few minutes before removing the skins.
2. Peel the carrots and cut off the tops. Chop them into cubes and steam them for 18 minutes or until they're soft. Allow the carrots to cool down after removing them from the steamer.
3. Combine the carrots, cumin, ground coriander, peeled garlic, 3 tbsp of olive oil, 1 cup of coconut flour, lemon juice, tahini paste, half of the chopped cilantro, and salt and pepper in a food processor. Scrape the sides of the processor and continue blending the ingredients until smooth. Stir the remainder of the chopped cilantro into the mixture.
4. Roll 1-inch balls with the mixture and cover them with sesame seeds. Line a baking tray with parchment paper and place them on the tray. Paint them with some olive oil. Pop your balls into the oven for 10 minutes. Remove them from the oven, flip

them over, and put them back into the oven to bake for an additional 10 minutes.
5. Remove your falafels from the oven, serve, and enjoy!

Dinner: Vegan Tikka Masala

Time: 35 minutes

Makes: 5 servings

Prep Time: 20 minutes

Cook Time: 15 minutes

Nutritional Value (per serving):

Net carbs	9g
Fat	21g
Protein	5g
Calories	248

Ingredients for the cauliflower:
- 1 head cauliflower, broken into small florets
- 1 tsp ground cumin
- 1 tsp garam masala
- ½ tsp cayenne pepper
- ½ tsp salt
- 1 tbsp olive oil

Ingredients for the sauce:

- 4 tbsp coconut oil
- ½ white onion, diced
- 2 cloves garlic, minced
- 1 tbsp ginger, minced
- 1 tbsp garam masala
- 1 ½ tsp paprika
- ½ tsp cayenne pepper
- ½ tsp salt
- 1 ½ cup crushed tomatoes
- ½ cup water
- ½ cup coconut cream
- ¼ cup minced cilantro

Directions:

1. While the oven is preheating to 225°F, put the cauliflower florets in a large bowl with the oil and spices and stir them well so that all of the florets are covered.
2. Line a baking tray with aluminum foil and spread the coated cauliflower florets evenly on the tray. Pop the tray into the oven for 30 minutes.
3. Warm up the coconut oil in a pan over medium-high heat and fry the onions, garlic, and ginger for 5 minutes. Then, add the garam masala, paprika, ground cumin, cayenne pepper, and salt. Fry everything for 30 seconds until fragrant. Add the tomatoes, water, and cream and reduce the heat to medium. Allow the mixture to cook for 10 minutes, stirring every now and then.
4. Once the cauliflower is done, add it to the spicy combination and stir it well. Serve your delicious curry dish with a dash of fresh cilantro on top.

Day 6

Breakfast (Optional): Cinnamon and Pecan Porridge

Time: 15 minutes

Makes: 2 servings

Prep Time: 5 minutes

Cook Time: 10 minutes

Nutritional Value (per serving):

Net carbs	*5g*
Fat	*51g*
Protein	*14g*
Calories	*582*

Ingredients:

- ¼ cup coconut milk
- ¾ cup unsweetened almond milk
- ¼ cup almond butter (toasted)
- 1 tbsp coconut oil or MCT oil

- 2 tbsp whole chia seeds
- 2 tbsp hemp seeds
- ¼ cup pecan nuts, chopped
- ¼ cup unsweetened toasted flaked coconut
- ½ tsp cinnamon
- 5 to 10 drops liquid stevia (optional)

Directions:

1. Combine the coconut oil, almond butter, almond milk, and coconut milk in a saucepan over medium heat and bring it to a simmer. Once hot, take the pan off the heat. Stir in the chia seeds, hemp seeds, chopped pecan nuts, and toasted coconut flakes. Make sure that you reserve some coconut for the topping.
2. Add the cinnamon and sweetener and mix well. Allow your porridge to rest for 5 minutes before serving with a topping of the remaining coconut. You can enjoy this dish hot or cold.

Lunch: Lemony Garlic Roasted Broccoli

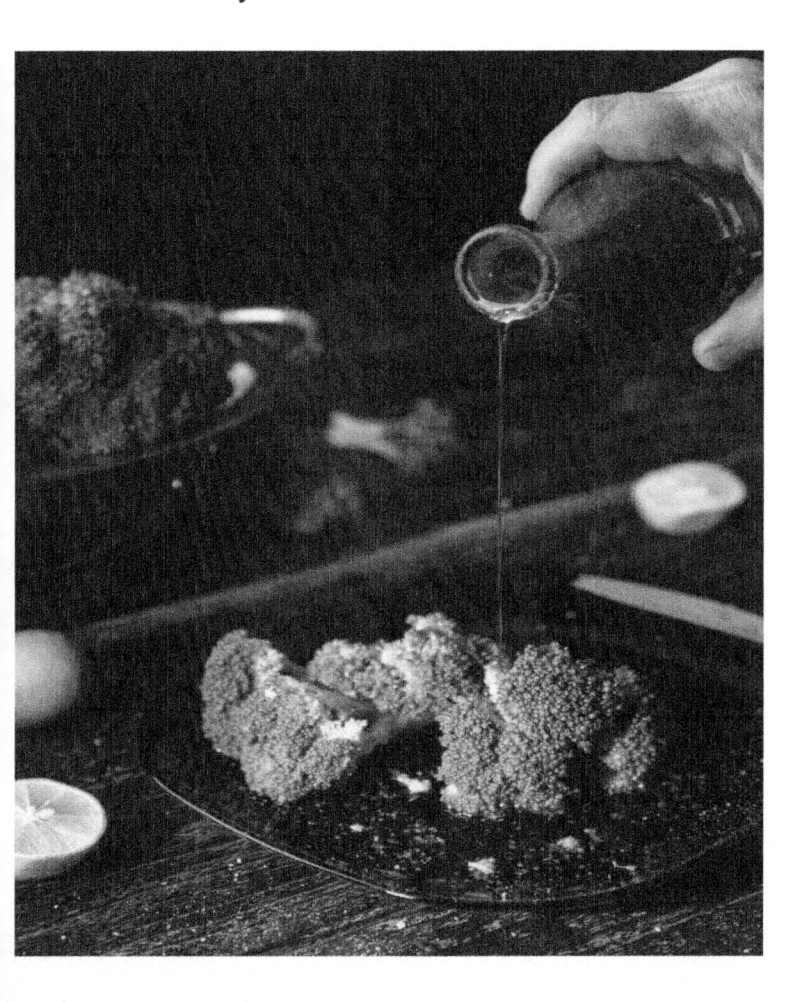

Time: 15 minutes

Makes: 4 servings

Prep Time: 5 minutes

Cook Time: 10 minutes

Nutritional Value (per serving):

Net carbs	7g
Fat	14g
Protein	4g
Calories	179

Ingredients:

- 2 medium heads broccoli, broken into florets
- ¼ cup olive oil
- 2 cloves garlic, minced
- 2 tbsp fresh lemon juice
- ½ tsp salt
- 1 tsp dried Italian herbs (topping)

Directions:

1. While the oven is preheating to 450°F, combine the minced garlic and olive oil.
2. On a large baking tray, spread out the broccoli florets evenly and drizzle them with your garlic olive oil mixture. Add a dash of fresh lemon juice and a pinch of salt to the broccoli and pop it into the oven for 12 to 15 minutes or until crispy and tender.
3. Remove the tray from the oven, add a dash of Italian herbs, and serve immediately.

Dinner: Pesto Zoodles (Zucchini Noodles)

Time: 15 minutes

Makes: 4 servings

Serving Size: 2 cups

Prep Time: 10 minutes

Cook Time: 5 minutes

Nutritional Value (per serving):

Net carbs	8g
Fat	42g
Protein	6g
Calories	452

Ingredients:
- 4 medium zucchinis, sliced into thin strips
- ½ cup pesto sauce
- 2 avocados
- 1 cup pitted kalamata olives
- ¼ cup sun-dried tomatoes, drained and sliced
- ¼ cup fresh basil
- 2 tbsp coconut oil or olive oil

- Salt to taste

Directions:
1. Spread the zoodles in a frying pan with coconut or olive oil and allow them to fry for 2 to 5 minutes or to your liking.
2. Peel, de-stone, and slice the avocados in half. Then, cut them into strips. Drain the olives and the sun-dried tomatoes.
3. Remove the zoodles from the stove and scoop pesto in. Stir it well and add a dash of salt.
4. Plate your zoodles and top them off with avocado, olives, tomatoes, and a dash of fresh basil. Serve immediately.

Day 7

Breakfast (Optional): Dairy-Free Ketoccino

Time: 5 minutes

Makes: 1 cup

Prep Time: 5 minutes

Nutritional Value (per serving):

Net carbs	2g
Fat	12g
Protein	1g
Calories	113

Ingredients:

- ⅓ cup espresso
- ¼ cup liquid coconut milk
- A pinch of cinnamon
- Sweetener to taste

Directions:

1. Prepare the espresso and shake the coconut milk for approximately 30 seconds before heating the required amount in the microwave until warm.
2. Pour the hot milk into the espresso, and hold back the foam with a spoon or a knife. When the cup is ⅔ full, top it with froth and a sprinkle of cinnamon.

Lunch: Spicy Zucchini Chips

Time: 1 hour and 15 minutes

Makes: 4 servings

Serving Size: ½ cup

Prep Time: 15 minutes

Cook Time: 1 hour

Nutritional Value (per serving):

Net carbs	*3g*
Fat	*4g*
Protein	*1g*
Calories	*54*

Ingredients:
- 2 medium zucchinis
- 1 lime, juiced, and zest
- 1 tbsp olive oil
- ½ tsp chili powder
- ½ tsp salt

Directions:

1. While the oven is preheating to 265°F, combine the chili powder, lime zest, and juice in a bowl.
2. Slice the zucchini as thinly as possible. Coat the slices with the chili powder mixture.
3. Place the zucchini slices on a lined baking tray and add a dash of salt and olive oil. Pop them in the oven for 45 to 60 minutes to crisp up.

Dinner: Spinach and Mushroom Soup

Time: 25 minutes

Makes: 4 servings

Serving Size: 1 cup

Prep Time: 10 minutes

Cook Time: 15 minutes

Nutritional Value (per serving):

Net carbs	8g
Fat	29g
Protein	7g
Calories	314

Ingredients:

- ¼ cup olive oil
- ½ onion, diced
- 1 lb brown mushrooms, sliced
- 2 cups vegetable stock
- 9 oz spinach
- ½ cup coconut cream (divided)
- Sea salt and ground pepper to taste

Directions:

1. In a large pot, heat the olive oil over medium heat and add the onions to fry until soft. Then, pour the mushrooms into the pot and allow it to cook for an additional 5 to 6 minutes.
2. Add the spinach and vegetable stock to the pot and bring it to a boil before reducing the heat. Let it simmer for 10 minutes.
3. Remove mixture from the heat and stir half of the coconut cream in. Allow it to cook for 2 minutes before using a stick blender to blend the mixture until smooth.
4. Serve with a dash of extra cream and enjoy!

Conclusion

To follow the keto diet successfully, you need to change your mindset. The biggest problem you might come across when reprogramming your mindset is the idea of eating fat to lose weight. We're so used to the idea that fat will have a negative impact on our health, but we need to get it out of our heads. Research has proven that fat is good for us. Starch is the real enemy; cutting starch out of our diet is the first step to leading a healthy lifestyle.

There is so much information available on the benefits of allowing your body to go into a state of ketosis. Change your idea of the keto diet. You will, in no way whatsoever, be starving yourself. In the beginning, it might be a challenge. Everything that is good for us is usually a challenge at first, though. Push through the beginning stages of keto and reap the results afterward. I promise you that it will get easier if you stick to it!

Develop a routine and try your best to follow that routine every day. The longer you do, the easier it gets! Naturally, setting goals for yourself is part of developing a routine. The keto diet is not just about losing weight. If your reason behind the keto diet is to lose weight, stick a picture of someone you admire to the fridge. This way, you're setting a weight-loss goal for yourself. If you're interested in the keto diet for its energy benefits, write down an exercise goal weekly (for example, I want to walk 10 miles this week), and stick it to your mirror. It can be as simple as wanting to wake up an hour earlier every morning to spend some time with your dog before you go to work. It is important, however, to be realistic.

This brings me to the next point; realistic goals are the key to perseverance! Setting goals for yourself that have nothing to do with who you are or what you prefer in life will not be easy to stick to. If you know that you don't like running, don't try it. If you're not built like a twig, don't set a goal for yourself to become one. Do you struggle to follow diets because you have a sweet tooth? Search for low-carb high-fat dessert recipes and enjoy them! You don't have to change anything about who you are to live a healthier lifestyle.

Stay motivated to stick to this diet by encouraging yourself daily. This really is as easy as sticking motivational quotes to anything around the house—a mirror, the front door, your fridge. You are awesome, and it's time that you build yourself up by adding some words of encouragement to your day as a reminder! Don't make the scale a priority; grab the measuring tape and bathe in your weight-loss achievements! Tap yourself on the shoulder for losing a few inches (even if it is less than you'd expected). Everyone's journey is not your journey; we're all unique. Your results cannot be compared with anyone else's. Celebrate the fact that you feel better, do more, eat less and live healthier!

You can still be the social butterfly you are. You don't have to isolate yourself when you start this diet. Enjoy the quality of restaurant food the keto way instead of saying no when your family or friends want to spend some time with you. Better yet, get one of them on board so that you're not alone! Eat the bun-less burger, have the whipped cream and strawberries for dessert, and enjoy a full-fat latte or cappuccino. You're not supposed to suffer on this diet; it requires nothing more than a few minor adjustments that will eventually become a habit. Besides, the delicious, flavorful recipes included in this guide are sure to make you feel satisfied and curb cravings!

If you're interested in starting with the keto diet, do it now. Never wait for things to calm down, speed up, or change. The more you postpone the greater the chances are that you're going to move on with your busy life and regret that you didn't start sooner. The best time to start is today.

References

2 Week Vegetarian Keto Diet Plan | KetoDiet Blog. (2015, July 5). KetoDiet. https://ketodietapp.com/Blog/lchf/2-week-vegetarian-keto-diet-plan#tips

3 Steps to a Successful Keto Mindset for Weight Loss on Keto. (2020, December 27). https://www.castleinthemountains.com/keto-mindset/

10 Health Benefits of Low-Carb and Ketogenic Diets. (2018, November 20). Healthline. https://www.healthline.com/nutrition/10-benefits-of-low-carb-ketogenic-diets#TOC_TITLE_HDR_2

15 Foods You Can't Eat on Keto (and What to Choose Instead) | Everyday Health. (n.d.). EverydayHealth.com. Retrieved March 10, 2021, from https://www.everydayhealth.com/ketogenic-diet/foods-you-can-t-eat-on-keto-and-what-to-choose-instead/

Aksungar, F. B., Topkaya, A. E., & Akyildiz, M. (2007). Interleukin-6, C-reactive protein and biochemical parameters during prolonged intermittent fasting. Annals of Nutrition & Metabolism, 51(1), 88–95. https://doi.org/10.1159/000100954

Albert, B. B., Derraik, J. G. B., Brennan, C. M., Biggs, J. B., Smith, G. C., Garg, M. L., Cameron-Smith, D., Hofman, P. L., & Cutfield, W. S. (2014). Higher omega-3 index is associated with increased insulin sensitivity and more favourable metabolic profile in middle-aged overweight men. Scientific Reports, 4(1). https://doi.org/10.1038/srep06697

Alcoholic beverage, beer, regular, all Nutrition Facts & Calories. (n.d.). Nutritiondata.self.com. https://nutritiondata.self.com/facts/beverages/3827/2

Alirezaei, M., Kemball, C. C., Flynn, C. T., Wood, M. R., Whitton, J. L., & Kiosses, W. B. (2010). Short-term fasting induces profound neuronal autophagy. Autophagy, 6(6), 702–710. https://doi.org/10.4161/auto.6.6.12376

B Keogh, J., & M Clifton, P. (2020). Energy intake and satiety responses of eggs for breakfast in overweight and obese adults—A crossover study. International Journal of Environmental Research and Public Health, 17(15), 5583. https://doi.org/10.3390/ijerph17155583

Barnosky, A. R., Hoddy, K. K., Unterman, T. G., & Varady, K. A. (2014). Intermittent fasting vs daily calorie restriction for type 2 diabetes prevention: a review of human findings. Translational Research, 164(4), 302–311. https://doi.org/10.1016/j.trsl.2014.05.013

Blackman, M. R. (2002). Growth hormone and sex steroid administration in healthy aged women and men. JAMA, 288(18), 2282. https://doi.org/10.1001/jama.288.18.2282

Bostock, E. C. S., Kirkby, K. C., Taylor, B. V., & Hawrelak, J. A. (2020). Consumer reports of "keto flu" associated with the ketogenic diet. Frontiers in Nutrition, 7. https://doi.org/10.3389/fnut.2020.00020

Calton, J. B. (2010). Prevalence of micronutrient deficiency in popular diet plans. Journal of the International Society of Sports Nutrition, 7(1). https://doi.org/10.1186/1550-2783-7-24

Capriles, V. D., & Arêas, J. a. G. (2016). Approaches to reduce the glycemic response of gluten-free products: in vivo and in vitro studies. Food & Function, 7(3), 1266–1272. https://doi.org/10.1039/c5fo01264c

Centers for Disease Control and Prevention. (2019). FastStats - Leading Causes of Death. CDC. https://www.cdc.gov/nchs/fastats/leading-causes-of-death.htm

Champ, C. E., Palmer, J. D., Volek, J. S., Werner-Wasik, M., Andrews, D. W., Evans, J. J., Glass, J., Kim, L., & Shi, W. (2014). Targeting metabolism with a ketogenic diet during the treatment of glioblastoma multiforme. Journal of Neuro-Oncology, 117(1), 125–131. https://doi.org/10.1007/s11060-014-1362-0

Chowdhury, R., Warnakula, S., Kunutsor, S., Crowe, F., Ward, H. A., Johnson, L., Franco, O. H., Butterworth, A. S., Forouhi, N. G., Thompson, S. G., Khaw, K.-T., Mozaffarian, D., Danesh, J., & Di Angelantonio, E. (2014). Association of dietary, circulating, and supplement fatty acids with coronary risk: a systematic review and meta-analysis. Annals of Internal Medicine, 160(6), 398–406. https://doi.org/10.7326/M13-1788

Cintineo, H. P., Arent, M. A., Antonio, J., & Arent, S. M. (2018). Effects of protein supplementation on performance and recovery in resistance and endurance training. Frontiers in Nutrition, 5(83). https://doi.org/10.3389/fnut.2018.00083

CISSN, A. H. and V. K., PhD, CSCS. (2020, January 13). The Complete Vegan Keto Diet and Food List. Onnit Academy. https://www.onnit.com/academy/vegan-keto-diet/

Cn, B., Cj, A., J, B., Js, V., & Ml, F. (2013, March 1). Whole egg consumption improves lipoprotein profiles and insulin sensitivity to a greater extent than yolk-free egg substitute in individuals with metabolic syndrome. Metabolism: Clinical and experimental. https://pubmed.ncbi.nlm.nih.gov/23021013/

Coffee linked to lower body fat in women: Compounds in coffee may have anti-obesity properties. (n.d.). ScienceDaily. Retrieved March 12, 2021, from https://www.sciencedaily.com/releases/2020/05/200513200402.htm

Collier, R. (2013). Intermittent fasting: the science of going without. Canadian Medical Association Journal, 185(9), E363–E364. https://doi.org/10.1503/cmaj.109-4451

Cooper, R., Naclerio, F., Allgrove, J., & Jimenez, A. (2012). Creatine supplementation with specific view to exercise/sports performance: an update. Journal of the International Society of Sports Nutrition, 9(1). https://doi.org/10.1186/1550-2783-9-33

Cotton, M. (2014). How Our Bodies Turn Food Into Energy. Kaiserpermanente.org. https://wa.kaiserpermanente.org/healthAndWellness?item=%2Fcommon%2FhealthAndWellness%2Fconditions%2Fdiabetes%2FfoodProcess.html

Crozier, S. J., Preston, A. G., Hurst, J. W., Payne, M. J., Mann, J., Hainly, L., & Miller, D. L. (2011). Cacao seeds are a "super fruit": A comparative analysis of various fruit powders and products. Chemistry Central Journal, 5(1), 5. https://doi.org/10.1186/1752-153x-5-5

D'Andrea Meira, I., Romão, T. T., Pires do Prado, H. J., Krüger, L. T., Pires, M. E. P., & da Conceição, P. O. (2019). Ketogenic diet and epilepsy: What we know so far. Frontiers in Neuroscience, 13. https://doi.org/10.3389/fnins.2019.00005

Daley, C. A., Abbott, A., Doyle, P. S., Nader, G. A., & Larson, S. (2010). A review of fatty acid profiles and antioxidant content in grass-fed and grain-fed beef. Nutrition Journal, 9(1). https://doi.org/10.1186/1475-2891-9-10

De Bont, R., & van Larebeke, N. (2004). Endogenous DNA damage in humans: A review of quantitative data. Mutagenesis, 19(3), 169–185. https://doi.org/10.1093/mutage/geh025

Dehghan, M., Mente, A., Zhang, X., Swaminathan, S., Li, W., Mohan, V., Iqbal, R., Kumar, R., Wentzel-Viljoen, E., Rosengren, A., Amma, L. I., Avezum, A., Chifamba, J., Diaz, R., Khatib, R., Lear, S., Lopez-Jaramillo, P., Liu, X., Gupta, R., & Mohammadifard, N. (2017). Associations of fats and carbohydrate intake with cardiovascular disease and mortality in 18 countries from five continents (PURE): a prospective cohort study. The Lancet, 390(10107), 2050–2062. https://doi.org/10.1016/s0140-6736(17)32252-3

Di Lorenzo, C., Coppola, G., Sirianni, G., & Pierelli, F. (2013). Short term improvement of migraine headaches during ketogenic diet: a prospective observational study in a dietician clinical setting. The Journal of Headache and Pain, 14(Suppl 1), P219. https://doi.org/10.1186/1129-2377-1-S14-P219

Diet Doctor — Making Low Carb and Keto Simple. (n.d.). Diet Doctor. Retrieved March 22, 2021, from https://dietdoctor.com

DiMeglio, D., & Mattes, R. (2000). Liquid versus solid carbohydrate: effects on food intake and body weight. International Journal of Obesity, 24(6), 794–800. https://doi.org/10.1038/sj.ijo.0801229

Evangeliou, A., Vlachonikolis, I., Mihailidou, H., Spilioti, M., Skarpalezou, A., Makaronas, N., Prokopiou, A., Christodoulou, P., Liapi-Adamidou, G., Helidonis, E., Sbyrakis, S., & Smeitink, J. (2003). Application of a ketogenic diet in children with autistic behavior: Pilot study. Journal of Child Neurology, 18(2), 113–118. https://doi.org/10.1177/08830738030180020501

Faris, M. A.-I. E., Kacimi, S., Al-Kurd, R. A., Fararjeh, M. A., Bustanji, Y. K., Mohammad, M. K., & Salem, M. L. (2012). Intermittent fasting during Ramadan attenuates proinflammatory cytokines and immune cells in healthy subjects. Nutrition Research, 32(12), 947–955. https://doi.org/10.1016/j.nutres.2012.06.021

Fernando, W. M. A. D. B., Martins, I. J., Goozee, K. G., Brennan, C. S., Jayasena, V., & Martins, R. N. (2015). The role of dietary coconut for the prevention and treatment of Alzheimer's disease: potential mechanisms of action. British Journal of Nutrition, 114(1), 1–14. https://doi.org/10.1017/s0007114515001452

Fj, M., Ws, Y., Ja, E., Rc, A., & Ec, W. (2007, January 1). The Effect of a Low-Carbohydrate Ketogenic Diet and a Low-Fat Diet on Mood, Hunger, and Other Self-Reported Symptoms. Obesity (Silver Spring, Md.) https://pubmed.ncbi.nlm.nih.gov/17228046/

FoodData Central. (n.d.). Fdc.nal.usda.gov. Retrieved March 10, 2021 from https://fdc.nal.usda.gov/fdc-app.html#/food details/783909/nutrients

Foods to Eat on a Ketogenic Diet. (2020, October 16). Healthline https://www.healthline.com/nutrition/ketogenic-diet-foods#TOC_TITLE_HDR_5

Free 28-Day Keto Meal Plan. (2018, November 26). Keto Summit https://ketosummit.com/free-keto-meal-plan/

G, S., N, R., H, M., & P, S. (2015). Modern diet and its impact on human health. Journal of Nutrition & Food Sciences, 05(06) https://doi.org/10.4172/2155-9600.1000430

Goodrick, C. L., Ingram, D. K., Reynolds, M. A., Freeman, J. R., & Cider, N. L. (1982). Effects of intermittent feeding upon growth and life span in rats. Gerontology, 28(4), 233–241 https://doi.org/10.1159/000212538

Guasch-Ferré, M., Liu, X., Malik, V. S., Sun, Q., Willett, W. C., Manson, J. E., Rexrode, K. M., Li, Y., Hu, F. B., & Bhupathiraju, S. N. (2017). Nut consumption and risk of cardiovascular disease. Journal of the American College of Cardiology, 70(20), 2519–2532 https://doi.org/10.1016/j.jacc.2017.09.035

Gunnars, K. (2016, August 16). 10 Evidence-Based Health Benefits of Intermittent Fasting. Healthline https://www.healthline.com/nutrition/10-health-benefits-of-intermittent-fasting

Gunnars, K. (2020, January 1). 6 popular ways to do intermittent fasting. Healthline. https://www.healthline.com/nutrition/6-ways-to-do-intermittent-fasting

Heilbronn, L. K., Civitarese, A. E., Bogacka, I., Smith, S. R., Hulver, M., & Ravussin, E. (2005). Glucose tolerance and skeletal muscle gene expression in response to alternate day fasting. Obesity Research, 13(3), 574–581. https://doi.org/10.1038/oby.2005.61

Ho, K. Y., Veldhuis, J. D., Johnson, M. L., Furlanetto, R., Evans, W. S., Alberti, K. G., & Thorner, M. O. (1988). Fasting enhances growth hormone secretion and amplifies the complex rhythms of growth hormone secretion in man. Journal of Clinical Investigation, 81(4), 968–975. https://www.ncbi.nlm.nih.gov/pmc/articles/PMC329619/

How to Follow a Low-Carb Vegan Meal Plan: 1,200 Calories. (n.d.). EatingWell. Retrieved March 14, 2021, from https://www.eatingwell.com/article/291329/how-to-follow-a-low-carb-vegan-meal-plan-1200-calories/

https://www.facebook.com/ruledme. (2019a, February 18). A Comprehensive Guide To The Vegan Ketogenic Diet | Ruled Me. Ruled Me. https://www.ruled.me/comprehensive-guide-vegan-ketogenic-diet/

https://www.facebook.com/ruledme. (2019b, June 18). Ketosis, Ketones, and How It All Works | Ruled Me. Ruled Me. https://www.ruled.me/ketosis-ketones-and-how-it-works/

https://www.facebook.com/WebMD. (2016, October 31). What Are Ketones and Their Tests? WebMD; WebMD. https://www.webmd.com/diabetes/ketones-and-their-tests

Jabekk, P. T., Moe, I. A., Meen, H. D., Tomten, S. E., & Høstmark, A. T. (2010). Resistance training in overweight women on a ketogenic diet conserved lean body mass while reducing body fat. Nutrition & Metabolism, 7(1), 17 https://doi.org/10.1186/1743-7075-7-17

Johnson, J. B., Summer, W., Cutler, R. G., Martin, B., Hyun, D.-H., Dixit, V. D., Pearson, M., Nassar, M., Tellejohan, R., Maudsley, S., Carlson, O., John, S., Laub, D. R., & Mattson, M. P. (2007). Alternate day calorie restriction improves clinical findings and reduces markers of oxidative stress and inflammation in overweight adults with moderate asthma. Free Radical Biology and Medicine, 42(5), 665–674. https://doi.org/10.1016/j.freeradbiomed.2006.12.005

Kephart, W., Pledge, C., Roberson, P., Mumford, P., Romero, M., Mobley, C., Martin, J., Young, K., Lowery, R., Wilson, J., Huggins, K., & Roberts, M. (2018). The three-month effects of a ketogenic diet on body composition, blood parameters, and performance metrics in crossfit trainees: A pilot study. Sports, 6(1), 1. https://doi.org/10.3390/sports6010001

Keto meal plan: Easy 7-day menu and diet tips. (2019, December 13). Www.medicalnewstoday.com. https://www.medicalnewstoday.com/articles/327309#tips

Keto Summit - Everything You Need For Ketogenic Diet Success. (n.d.). Keto Summit. Retrieved March 22, 2021, from https://ketosummit.com

Ketogenic Diet 101: A Beginner's Guide. (n.d.). EatingWell. Retrieved March 11, 2021, from https://www.eatingwell.com/article/290697/ketogenic-diet-101-a-beginners-guide/

Kim, D. Y., Hao, J., Liu, R., Turner, G., Shi, F.-D., & Rho, J. M. (2012). Inflammation-mediated memory dysfunction and effects of a ketogenic diet in a murine model of multiple sclerosis. PloS One, 7(5), e35476. https://doi.org/10.1371/journal.pone.0035476

Klepper, J., Scheffer, H., Leiendecker, B., Gertsen, E., Binder, S., Leferink, M., Hertzberg, C., Näke, A., Voit, T., & Willemsen, M. A. (2005). Seizure control and acceptance of the ketogenic diet in GLUT1 deficiency syndrome: a 2- to 5-year follow-up of 15 children enrolled prospectively. Neuropediatrics, 36(5), 302–308. https://doi.org/10.1055/s-2005-872843

Krikorian, R., Shidler, M. D., Dangelo, K., Couch, S. C., Benoit, S. C., & Clegg, D. J. (2012). Dietary ketosis enhances memory in mild cognitive impairment. Neurobiology of Aging, 33(2), 425.e19–425.e27. https://doi.org/10.1016/j.neurobiolaging.2010.10.006

Kubala, J. (2018, November 5). Intermittent Fasting and Keto: Should You Combine the Two? Healthline. https://www.healthline.com/nutrition/intermittent-fasting-and-keto#should-you

Kuebler, U., Arpagaus, A., Meister, R. E., von Känel, R., Huber, S., Ehlert, U., & Wirtz, P. H. (2016). Dark chocolate attenuates intracellular pro-inflammatory reactivity to acute psychosocial stress in men: A randomized controlled trial. Brain, Behavior, and Immunity, 57, 200–208. https://doi.org/10.1016/j.bbi.2016.04.006

Laessle, R. G., Platte, P., Schweiger, U., & Pirke, K. M. (1996). Biological and psychological correlates of intermittent dieting behavior in young women. A model for bulimia nervosa. Physiology & Behavior, 60(1), 1–5. https://doi.org/10.1016/0031-9384(95)02215-5

Larbah, H. (2020, January 18). A 7-Day Vegan Keto Meal Plan That's Totally Doable. POPSUGAR Fitness. https://www.popsugar.com/fitness/Vegan-Keto-Meal-Plan-45066231

Lee, Y., Berryman, C. E., West, S. G., Chen, C. -Y. O., Blumberg, J. B., Lapsley, K. G., Preston, A. G., Fleming, J. A., & Kris-Etherton, P. M. (2017). Effects of dark chocolate and almonds on cardiovascular risk factors in overweight and obese individuals:

A randomized controlled-feeding trial. Journal of the American Heart Association, 6(12). https://doi.org/10.1161/jaha.116.005162

Lk, H., Sr, S., Ck, M., Sd, A., & E, R. (2005, January 1). Alternate-day Fasting in Nonobese Subjects: Effects on Body Weight, Body Composition, and Energy Metabolism. The American Journal of Clinical Nutrition. https://pubmed.ncbi.nlm.nih.gov/15640462/

Ltd, C. (n.d.). The ultimate low-carb diet app | Keto Diet App. KetoDiet. Retrieved March 22, 2021, from https://ketodietapp.com

Manninen, A. H. (2006). Very-low-carbohydrate diets and preservation of muscle mass. Nutrition & Metabolism, 3(1). https://doi.org/10.1186/1743-7075-3-9

Martin, B., Mattson, M. P., & Maudsley, S. (2006). Caloric restriction and intermittent fasting: Two potential diets for successful brain aging. Ageing Research Reviews, 5(3), 332–353. https://doi.org/10.1016/j.arr.2006.04.002

Mavropoulos, J., Yancy, W., Hepburn, J., & Westman, E. (2005). The effects of a low carbohydrate, ketogenic diet on the polycystic ovary syndrome: A pilot story. Nutrition & Metabolism, 2(1), 35. https://doi.org/10.1186/1743-7075-2-35

Mawer, R. (2020, October 22). The Ketogenic Diet: A Detailed Beginner's Guide to Keto. Healthline. https://www.healthline.com/nutrition/ketogenic-diet-101#tips

McCarty, M. F., & DiNicolantonio, J. J. (2016). Lauric acid-rich medium-chain triglycerides can substitute for other oils in cooking applications and may have limited pathogenicity. Open Heart, 3(2), e000467. https://doi.org/10.1136/openhrt-2016-000467

Migala, J. (n.d.-a). 10 Steps Beginners Should Take Before Trying the Keto Diet | Everyday Health. EverydayHealth.com. https://www.everydayhealth.com/diet-nutrition/ketogenic-diet/steps-beginners-should-take-before-trying-keto-diet/

Migala, J. (n.d.-b). 15 Burning Questions About the Keto Diet, Answered | Everyday Health. EverydayHealth.com. Retrieved March 5, 2021, from https://www.everydayhealth.com/ketogenic-diet/diet/burning-questions-about-keto-diet-answered/

Migala, J. (2019, August 23). What Are the Benefits and Risks of the Keto Diet? | Everyday Health. EverydayHealth.com. https://www.everydayhealth.com/diet-nutrition/ketogenic-diet/what-are-benefits-risks-keto-diet/

Moro, T., Tinsley, G., Bianco, A., Marcolin, G., Pacelli, Q. F., Battaglia, G., Palma, A., Gentil, P., Neri, M., & Paoli, A. (2016). Effects of eight weeks of time-restricted feeding (16/8) on basal metabolism, maximal strength, body composition, inflammation, and cardiovascular risk factors in resistance-trained males. Journal of Translational Medicine, 14(1). https://doi.org/10.1186/s12967-016-1044-0

Mychasiuk, R., & Rho, J. M. (2016). Genetic modifications associated with ketogenic diet treatment in the BTBRT+Tf/Jmouse model of autism spectrum disorder. Autism Research, 10(3), 456–471. https://doi.org/10.1002/aur.1682

Nebeling, L. C., Miraldi, F., Shurin, S. B., & Lerner, E. (1995). Effects of a ketogenic diet on tumor metabolism and nutritional status in pediatric oncology patients: two case reports. Journal of the American College of Nutrition, 14(2), 202–208. https://doi.org/10.1080/07315724.1995.10718495

Norgren, J., Sindi, S., Sandebring-Matton, A., Kåreholt, I., Daniilidou, M., Akenine, U., Nordin, K., Rosenborg, S., Ngandu, T., & Kivipelto, M. (2020). Ketosis after intake of coconut oil and caprylic acid—With and without glucose: A cross-over study in healthy older adults. Frontiers in Nutrition, 7 https://doi.org/10.3389/fnut.2020.00040

Phelps, J. R., Siemers, S. V., & El-Mallakh, R. S. (2013). The ketogenic diet for type II bipolar disorder. Neurocase, 19(5), 423–426 https://doi.org/10.1080/13554794.2012.690421

Phinney, S. D. (2004). Ketogenic diets and physical performance Nutrition & Metabolism, 1(1), 2 https://doi.org/10.1186/1743-7075-1-2

Rahal, A., Kumar, A., Singh, V., Yadav, B., Tiwari, R., Chakraborty, S., & Dhama, K. (2014, January 23). Oxidative Stress, Prooxidants and Antioxidants: The Interplay. BioMed Research International. https://www.hindawi.com/journals/bmri/2014/761264/

Reboredo-Rodríguez, P., Varela-López, A., Forbes-Hernández, T. Y., Gasparrini, M., Afrin, S., Cianciosi, D., Zhang, J., Manna, P. P., Bompadre, S., Quiles, J. L., Battino, M., & Giampieri, F. (2018) Phenolic compounds isolated from olive oil as nutraceutical tools for the prevention and management of cancer and cardiovascular diseases. International Journal of Molecular Sciences, 19(8). https://doi.org/10.3390/ijms19082305

Romani, A., Ieri, F., Urciuoli, S., Noce, A., Marrone, G., Nediani, C., & Bernini, R. (2019). Health effects of phenolic compounds found in extra-virgin olive oil, by-products, and leaf of olea europaea L. Nutrients, 11(8) https://doi.org/10.3390/nu11081776

Rusu, M. E., Simedrea, R., Gheldiu, A.-M., Mocan, A., Vlase, L., Popa D.-S., & Ferreira, I. C. F. R. (2019). Benefits of tree nut consumption on aging and age-related diseases: Mechanisms of actions. Trends in Food Science & Technology, 88, 104–120 https://doi.org/10.1016/j.tifs.2019.03.006

Smith, J., Rho, J. M., & Teskey, G. C. (2016). Ketogenic diet restores aberrant cortical motor maps and excitation-to-inhibition imbalance in the BTBR mouse model of autism spectrum disorder. Behavioural Brain Research, 304, 67–70. https://doi.org/10.1016/j.bbr.2016.02.015

Spritzler, F. (2016, September 12). 15 Health Conditions That May Benefit From a Ketogenic Diet. Healthline. https://www.healthline.com/nutrition/15-conditions-benefit-ketogenic-diet#TOC_TITLE_HDR_3

Storoni, M., & Plant, G. T. (2015). The therapeutic potential of the ketogenic diet in treating progressive multiple sclerosis. Multiple Sclerosis International, 2015, 1–9. https://doi.org/10.1155/2015/681289

Stubbs, B. J., Cox, P. J., Evans, R. D., Santer, P., Miller, J. J., Faull, O. K., Magor-Elliott, S., Hiyama, S., Stirling, M., & Clarke, K. (2017). On the metabolism of exogenous ketones in humans. Frontiers in Physiology, 8. https://doi.org/10.3389/fphys.2017.00848

Sussman, D., van Eede, M., Wong, M. D., Adamson, S. L., & Henkelman, M. (2013). Effects of a ketogenic diet during pregnancy on embryonic growth in the mouse. BMC Pregnancy and Childbirth, 13(1). https://doi.org/10.1186/1471-2393-13-109

Thorning, T. K., Raziani, F., Bendsen, N. T., Astrup, A., Tholstrup, T., & Raben, A. (2015). Diets with high-fat cheese, high-fat meat, or carbohydrate on cardiovascular risk markers in overweight postmenopausal women: a randomized crossover trial. The American Journal of Clinical Nutrition, 102(3), 573–581. https://doi.org/10.3945/ajcn.115.109116

Tikoo, K., Tripathi, D. N., Kabra, D. G., Sharma, V., & Gaikwad, A. B. (2007). Intermittent fasting prevents the progression of type I diabetic nephropathy in rats and changes the expression of Sir2 and p53. FEBS Letters, 581(5), 1071–1078. https://doi.org/10.1016/j.febslet.2007.02.006

Top 18 low-carb and keto controversies. (n.d.). Diet Doctor. Retrieved March 3, 2021, from https://www.dietdoctor.com/low carb/controversies

Tremblay, A., Doyon, C., & Sanchez, M. (2015). Impact of yogurt on appetite control, energy balance, and body composition. Nutrition Reviews, 73(suppl 1), 23–27. https://doi.org/10.1093/nutrit/nuv015

Tzur, A., Roberts, B., & Leaf, A. (2017, October 25). The Ketogenic Diet's Impact on Body Fat, Muscle Mass, Strength, and Endurance • Sci-Fit. Sci-Fit. https://sci-fit.net/ketogenic-diet fat-muscle-performance/

Varady, K. A., Bhutani, S., Church, E. C., & Klempel, M. C. (2009). Short-term modified alternate-day fasting: a novel dietary strategy for weight loss and cardioprotection in obese adults. The American Journal of Clinical Nutrition, 90(5), 1138–1143. https://doi.org/10.3945/ajcn.2009.28380

Veech, R. L. (2004). The therapeutic implications of ketone bodies: the effects of ketone bodies in pathological conditions: ketosis ketogenic diet, redox states, insulin resistance, and mitochondrial metabolism. Prostaglandins, Leukotrienes and Essential Fatty Acids, 70(3), 309–319. https://doi.org/10.1016/j.plefa.2003.09.007

Wang, L., Bordi, P. L., Fleming, J. A., Hill, A. M., & Kris-Etherton, P. M. (2015). Effect of a moderate fat diet with and without avocados on lipoprotein particle number, size and subclasses in overweight and obese ddults: A randomized, controlled trial. Journal of the American Heart Association: Cardiovascular and Cerebrovascular Disease, 4(1). https://doi.org/10.1161/JAHA.114.001355

West, D., Abou Sawan, S., Mazzulla, M., Williamson, E., & Moore, D. (2017). Whey protein supplementation enhances whole body protein metabolism and performance recovery after resistance exercise: A Double-Blind crossover study. Nutrients, 9(7), 735. https://doi.org/10.3390/nu9070735

Wnuk, A. (n.d.). How do ketogenic diets help people with epilepsy? Www.brainfacts.org. Retrieved March 8, 2021, from https://www.brainfacts.org/ic-diets-help-people-with-epilepsy-081418#:~:text=The%20ketogenic%20diet%20reduces%20the

www.3in1keto.com

Yancy, W. S., Foy, M., Chalecki, A. M., Vernon, M. C., & Westman, E. C. (2005). A low-carbohydrate, ketogenic diet to treat type 2 diabetes. Nutrition & Metabolism, 2(1), 34. https://doi.org/10.1186/1743-7075-2-34

Zhu, Y., Yan, Y., Gius, D. R., & Vassilopoulos, A. (2013). Metabolic regulation of sirtuins upon fasting and the implication for cancer. Current Opinion in Oncology, 25(6), 630–636. https://doi.org/10.1097/01.cco.0000432527.49984.a3

Zick, S. M., Snyder, D., & Abrams, D. I. (2018, November 15). Pros and cons of dietary strategies popular among cancer patients. Cancer Network. https://www.cancernetwork.com/view/dietary-strategies-cancer

Zuccoli, G., Marcello, N., Pisanello, A., Servadei, F., Vaccaro, S., Mukherjee, P., & Seyfried, T. N. (2010). Metabolic management of glioblastoma multiforme using standard therapy together with a restricted ketogenic diet: Case Report. Nutrition & Metabolism, 7(1), 33. https://doi.org/10.1186/1743-7075-7-33

Images

https://pixabay.com/get/g9cca22eedece792f2ceb576122c13277f0732d97bc98f9a8a295eb23b8298034e1d01fab991635bb556ddab35328d856_1280.jpg?attachment=

https://pixabay.com/get/gd6a412c36198521a309f496245b72b580a392d41239d8d60a83e88986b986d73209a6d84fa204ef4ac20cc50add8a257_640.jpg?attachment=

https://images.unsplash.com/photo-1613119719948-d53865658a88?ixlib=rb-1.2.1&q=80&fm=jpg&crop=entropy&cs=tinysrgb&dl=aneta-voborilova-aFqKIFZ-Idg-unsplash.jUnsplash.com.
https://images.unsplash.com/photo-1601823281975-75d81b28c373?ixlib=rb-1.2.1&q=80&fm=jpg&crop=entropy&cs=tinysrgb&dl=big-dodzy-sRAsn4cv1HI-unsplash.jpgpg

https://images.unsplash.com/photo-1558303420-f814d8a590f5?ixlib=rb-1.2.1&q=80&fm=jpg&crop=entropy&cs=tinysrgb&dl=roberto-martinez-iHgBWWFGrtY-unsplash.jpg&w=640

https://images.unsplash.com/photo-1492683962492-deef0ec456c0?ixlib=rb-1.2.1&q=80&fm=jpg&crop=entropy&cs=tinysrgb&dl=toa-heftiba-MSxw2vpQzx4-unsplash.jpg&w=640

https://images.unsplash.com/photo-1578859318509-62790b079366?ixlib=rb-1.2.1&q=80&fm=jpg&crop=entropy&cs=tinysrgb&dl=samee-anderson-x4l4U-pHF9s-unsplash.jpg&w=640

https://images.unsplash.com/photo-1584587727565-a486d45d58b4?ixlib=rb-1.2.1&q=80&fm=jpg&crop=entropy&cs=tinysrgb&dl=lyfe-fuel-_82CV9I-TP8-unsplash.jpg

https://images.unsplash.com/photo-1546241072-48010ad2862c?ixlib=rb-

.2.1&q=80&fm=jpg&crop=entropy&cs=tinysrgb&dl=sam-hojati-M4hazNIyTsk-unsplash.jpg&w=640

https://burst.shopifycdn.com/photos/healthy-dining-salads-wraps-and-bowls.jpg?width=4460&height=4460&exif=1&iptc=1&attachment=healthy-dining-salads-wraps-and-bowls.jpg

Printed in Great Britain
by Amazon